Coaches' Corner

Essays on Athletic Development, Coaching and Teaching.

JAMES MARSHALL

DEDICATION

Thanks to all the athletes I have coached, young and old, novice and experienced. I have learnt something from all of you.

Thanks to all the coaches who have helped me along the way, especially Keith Morgan OBE at Crystal Palace Weightlifting who helped me when I was in a dark place with Karate and showed me the light.

Thanks to all my GAIN colleagues for sharing, teaching and inspiring me to become a better version of myself.

CONTENTS

Chapter		Page
	Dedication	iii
	Foreword: Brian McCormick	vii
	Preface	1
1	Redefining Physical Education post-Covid	4
2	Structural Integrity	9
3	A Note on Session Design	12
4	How to Stem the Mini-Band Epidemic	13
5	What is Athletic Development?	16
6	Long and Strong: Posture Redefined	19
7	Teaching Children How to Move	23
8	Managing the Time	27
9	Tenets of Speed Development	29
10	How to Make Your Team Faster	32
11	What is Physical Literacy?	36
12	Are You Recovering Well Enough?	40
13	Sports Science for Coaches	43
14	Intention and Attention	46
15	Creating Your Own Sporting Culture	49
16	How to Create a World Class Physical Education Programme	52
17	Core Training For Children	57
18	Helping Your Athletes Decide	62

19   Teaching Games in Primary School   65

20   A Million Sporty Girls Drop Out of Sport   70

21   Coaching With Compassion or For   73
     Compliance

22   Three Dimensional Agility   76

23   Movement is the Foundation of Sports   79
     Injury Rehabilitation

24   Reducing Football Hamstring Injuries   82

25   Sprint Training for Children   85

26   Mental Health in Adolescent Athletes   89

27   Reflective Practice for Sports Coaches   93

28   Seven Sports Science Myths   99

29   Micro-Dosing for Efficiency   103

30   Why PE Should be More 'We' Than 'Me'   107

31   A Simple Guide to Developing Powerful   110
     Athletes

32   Are You Teaching or Testing?   115

33   Individualisation in Group Environments   118

34   Don't be Cruel to Kittens (Or Children)   121

35   Improve Your Coaching Through   125
     Storytelling

36   From Textbook to Notebook   127

37   Sore or Injured?   133

38   A Five Step Plan to Cure Insomnia   136

39   The Quest for Ultra-Performance   143

40 Play, Play and Play   146

41 Beware the Volume Trap   149

42 The Dangers of Labelling Youth Athletes   156

43 How to Handle a Losing Streak   159

44 The Oxymoronic Talent Pathway   162

45 The Three Stages of Fitness Testing   167

46 Creating Frankenstein's Monster in the Gym   171

47 A Movement Manifesto   173

48 Go Hard, Go Fast, Finish it, Go Again   176

49 How to Make Pre-Season Training   181
    Interesting, Relevant and Fun

50 Exercise as Medicine   185

51 Weightlifting for Juniors   189

52 What Is The End Game For Your Athletes?   191

FOREWORD

I am honored to write the foreword to Coaches' Corner because James Marshall epitomizes the 21st Century coach, an old-school approach based on the experiences of a veteran athlete and coach informed by a curiosity to integrate the latest research to create a great environment for all interested athletes.

I met James at GAIN, Vern Gambetta's athletic development conference, as he led morning practical sessions focused on developing athleticism and coordination.

He is a coaches' coach, expertly explaining and teaching the fundamentals of movement. James is a voracious reader and published novelist, but despite his fondness for the written word, his straightforward reflections on coaching, physical education, talent development, and more provide accessible lessons rather than obfuscating with flowery language and pseudoscientific rhetoric with little to no actual explication or practicality.

Coaching once was fairly simple, as a person used his or her accumulated knowledge and experience to assist others in their athletic pursuits, possibly integrating some studies into foundational sciences such as biomechanics, physiology, and psychology. Physical education was broad and general and focused on health and physical activity, developing competence in basic movements eventually leading to more complex sports skills.

Of course, in our infinite wisdom, we over complicated coaching and de-emphasized physical education. Coaches' Corner addresses many of the lessons we lost in our rush to specialize and perform.

I hesitate in my descriptions, as simple and old school have a negative connotation, especially within sports where everyone chases the new and advanced, pivoting year by year to follow the latest fad advertised as the way. I use simple and old school as the greatest possible compliment, an acknowledgment of James' ability to infuse his coaching and writing with easily actionable steps leading toward improvement and success without complicating his writing with gobbledygook.

Albert Einstein famously said, "If you can't explain it to a six-year-old, you don't understand it yourself." James explains complicated and complex topics and movements simply, enabling beginners and experts to understand and use the information. His approach is old school in that he emphasizes the major movement fundamentals in athletics, gymnastics, and weightlifting. These provide a foundation for continued exposure to the specific sports, for a healthy, active lifestyle, or to transfer to other sports. The passages are backed by James' years of experience as a coach, teacher, gym owner, and athlete.

Like Gambetta and Dan John, James conveys simple, uncomplicated, but impactful wisdom. Whether writing about talent development pathways, mental health, exercising goals with a busy schedule, or improving posture for performance, he has lived the lessons, which coaches and athletes can use immediately to improve their learning and performance.

This collection is written by a true practitioner, based on years of experience, but infused with current research to supplement and support his practice and coaching. Simple and old school do not mean stuck in one's ways and never-changing, but a solid, evolving foundation from which to explain complex concepts for a general audience. Marshall is a master at his craft, and his expertise comes forth through these passages.

Brian McCormick PhD.

PREFACE

When I was at school in the 1980s, we hadn't heard of the words 'academy' or 'talent.' Physical education was regular and robust, with two lessons a week where we wore white t-shirts, and one 'Games' lesson a week where we wore thick, reversible long-sleeved cotton shirts for football, rugby and hockey for two terms. We were allowed to wear white T-shirts in the summer term for athletics, tennis and cricket.

At lunchtimes, we played tag, 'forty-forty', leapfrog, football plus other games like hurling ourselves down grass banks to see if we could survive, throwing tennis balls to boys and girls from the other class in our year over portacabins and epic snowball wars.

When we got home, we played outside on our estate until it got dark: boys and girls, both younger and older than us.

A few kids disappeared on occasion to go to a tennis club, or a cricket club and one boy did judo. These were the exceptions. There was no pathway (except the ones to the recreation ground) and no adult telling us what to do.

I thought, because we had no money, I was unlucky in my childhood for not receiving extra coaching. And yet, when I look at the landscape today, I realise how lucky I was. I was allowed to play without inhibition, to sample many different sports thanks to our p.e. teachers, and to create games of our choosing, playing against our friends.

Now, many teachers (and fewer policymakers) don't understand the difference between p.e. and sport, children are ferried from one organised activity to another, with green spaces, parks and cycle paths vanishing over the decades. Parents are pressured into paying for private tuition for their children so they don't 'fall behind' or spend so much time on their phones that they don't play catch or football or French cricket with their children.

And that's before the Sports National Governing Bodies (NGBs) get involved.

I worked in health and fitness clubs for eight years before starting my MSc in sports coaching. I then spent 10 years working as a fitness coach for sports teams and schools, gaining 'strength and conditioning' qualifications along the way. This included working with age-group National and Regional squads in rugby union and league, volleyball, fencing, golf and visually impaired football.

Something was wrong. What I'd learnt from the textbooks or the lecturers did not correlate with what I saw with my own eyes and learned from my own experiences. The young people being thrust into these training environments were simply unable to cope with the pressures of training. They were highly specialised in one sport and had some skill, but their physical movement was limited.

I had two lightbulb moments within one year (2009).

First, I attended a day's workshop with Kelvin Giles. Kelvin took us through his Physical Competency Assessment (PCA) and explained how basic movements needed to be mastered before more complex movements could be learned.
This was different from the 'Max-effort' battery of fitness tests that were deemed 'necessary' to measure athletes by NGBs and Lecturers alike.

Second, I met Paula Jardine who headed up the 'South West Talent' programme, funded by Sport England. Paula invited me to work with the programme and the group of athletes they were selected from all sports. Paula had an excellent knowledge of the theory of Long-Term Athlete Development (LTAD) and was looking for practitioners to help her implement it.

Together, over the next two years, we helped dozens of young people get better, in a multi-disciplinary environment where coaches, athletes, parents, physiotherapists, Paula and myself shared information and ideas and fed them back into the programme.

Paula explained that my childhood background, instead of being disadvantaged, was near to ideal in terms of rich, varied learning opportunities.

My two children, Daisy and Jack, were born just before this programme started. Watching them grow and develop added a new understanding of movement and learning.

I attended the first of nine of Vern Gambetta's GAIN conferences in 2011 and my eyes opened wider. Here was a group of world-class practitioners: S&C coaches, physiotherapists, track and field coaches, athletic trainers and p.e. teachers, gathered together to share and learn. The early morning 'Movement Madness' sessions gave me the practical tools to do my job that my MSc and other qualifications had failed to provide. I use those tools every day in my coaching.

My knowledge and enthusiasm knew no bounds, the athletes I worked with were thriving and the parents were on board. And yet, I felt constrained by the NGBs who insisted on S&C coaches working in silos and providing test results to feed into their data banks, rather than looking at the sports performance and injury reduction.

It was then that I decided to set up my club. A place where local children could come and train in a few key disciplines and learn to move and explore and get fit in a safe and fun environment.

Excelsior Athletic Development Club was born in Willand ten years ago, in 2014.

I gained further qualifications in gymnastics, athletics and weightlifting and now coach all three sports. My children attended the club and became competent movers, able to pick up sports at school and compete when they wanted. They also did horse riding, indoor climbing and life-saving with other excellent, local coaches.

I helped our Parish Council turn barren fields into parks with a variety of playground equipment for children to play on for free and picnic benches for parents to rest upon. They have since added a BMX pump track and a skateboard ramp: all free to use and within our village.

I was never 'Good' at sports at school: I was the youngest child in the school year (and the smallest for a long time). I played a lot and represented the school in hockey, football and rugby.

This book contains a series of essays and articles that expand on my knowledge and experiences referenced above. Some of what you read will be familiar, some will turn 'perceived wisdom' on its head. The essays are my best effort at the moment of writing.

Everything I write is designed to help teachers, coaches and parents improve their practice so that the children in their care can benefit.

Children deserve the best we can give them.

1: REDEFINING PHYSICAL EDUCATION POST-COVID

As pupils returned to school after the many lockdowns, they found that the opportunities to play team sports were reduced. Physical distancing meant that rugby, football and netball, for example, were too difficult to administer. Travelling between schools was also reduced: the risk of transferring the virus was too high.

Instead of P.E. Departments floundering without their Adult-led competitive sports fixtures and syllabi, there was an opportunity for schools to return to traditional physical education and prioritise the health and well-being of the pupils.
Teachers could teach, rather than referee or organise fixtures, and inspire a generation of young people to become physically active rather than slavishly follow the crowd and watch young people disengage from physical activity.

As the Japanese proverb says,
"The barn burned down/ now I can see the moon."

Instead of trying to copy what 'elite' sports do, there was a chance to refocus on the needs, wants and desires of our children. We can bring joy and challenge and inspiration and expression back into the minds and bodies of these young people.

In this essay I shall lay out the following ideas:
· Debunking the Traditional Sports Myth
· The Health of the Nation and how elitism has infected the state school syllabus.
· How P.E., can taught well in Primary Schools.

Why 'Traditional Sports' are not traditional

Many teachers refer to rugby and cricket as 'Traditional sports' versus 'new-age' sports like Parkour. This has become part of the P.E. vernacular and is rarely challenged.

I challenge this misconception and blame Thomas Hughes.

Hughes wrote 'Tom Brown's Schooldays', the popular nineteenth-century novel that shows the character-building effects of rough games and cricket on boys like Tom, at Rugby school. Pierre de Coubertin (founder of the modern Olympics) was a fan of the book and it formed part of his premise for recreating the Modern Games.

Thomas Arnold, the real Head Master of Rugby School (The Doctor in TBS) was no sporting evangelist, he preferred the curing of souls and the developing of boys' intellects. His educational reforms and treatises did not advocate sport. So, it is the fictionalised account of Rugby School, aided by William Webb Ellis picking up the ball (1823) and running with it, that has influenced our culture. Rugby School, for those that don't know, is an Independent (fee-paying) school.

Parkour is often referred to as 'non-traditional' yet it predates rugby. Whereas in Britain the playing fields of Eton were credited for defeating Napoleon at Waterloo, in Germany it was boys playing in the woods. Scared by the prospect of invasion by Napoleon, Father Jahn took a group of boys into the woods outside Berlin, where they practised running, jumping and leaping over and up obstacles. When the winter came, they moved indoors and built apparatus that simulated the outdoor obstacles. So began modern gymnastics.

Gymnastics, wrestling, weight-lifting and boxing were all included in the Ancient Games. They are more 'Traditional' than team sports and yet have disappeared from school curricula: why not bring them back now?

The Health of the Nation and how elitism has infected the state school syllabus

Twelve years ago the UK hosted the Olympics and boasted of a legacy to inspire generations to follow. There was no evidence from previous countries that any uptake in physical activity followed their hosting of the Olympics.

The UK invested £14.8 billion so that 80,000 people could sit in a stadium to watch a few people run around a track. In the case of the women's 1500m final, 6 of the 9 top finishers were associated with taking Performance-enhancing Enhancing Drugs. It has been called, 'the dirtiest race in history.'

West Ham United now uses the stadium, so the UK taxpayer has helped subsidise a professional football club's business. The clamour to be at the top of the medals table has resulted in millions of pounds being invested to support a few individuals in achieving their dreams. Funding for sports in the UK has been dependent on their achieving medal success for years now. UK Sport has deliberately targeted fewer sports that can offer 'better returns' since the GB team had poor results in Atlanta in 1996.

The UK is famous for winning medals sitting down and going backwards: sailing, rowing, cycling and equestrian. Expensive sports to take up so fewer countries have participants which increases the UK's chances of winning. Team GB does less well at weight lifting, athletics and swimming, sports which rely less on technology and so equalising the odds.

Investment has been diverted from 'grassroots' to 'performance' to showcase 'our talent'. For example, Modern Pentathlon received £6,140,529 between 2017 and 2020 on the back of winning a silver medal in 2012. Basketball, which has zero chance of winning a medal at the Olympics, has received no funding.

According to The Independent (2016), basketball was second only to football with 218,000 children aged 14-16 playing the sport once a week.

How many children were inspired to take up modern pentathlon after its lone medal in 2012? The money invested in Team GB is mind-blowing: for Rio, it was £274,465,541. When you realise that of the 96 gold medals won by Team GB between Atlanta (1996) and Rio (2016) just 12 people won or contributed to 49 of them, you can then think, "How has this helped the country?"

When governments say that investing in sports and the Olympics is good for the country, what they mean is that it is good for a tiny minority of athletes and a lot of support staff.

The Olympics was a smokescreen that covered the underlying poor health of our nation. I wrote to my local MP, Neil 'Tractor Porn' Parish, in 2011 to ask him about investment in school Physical Education. He wrote back and mentioned the Olympics as inspiring a generation.

Twelve years on, and how has that worked out? The Prime Minister, who was Mayor of London at the time of the Olympics was hardly inspired: he weighed 110kg and only his hospitalisation from COVID made him think about losing weight. His poor health inspired him to do something, not taking selfies with Gold Medal winners.

The obsession with 'winning' has infected our state school physical education system. Now there is a narrow syllabus and the focus is on replicating adult sports with their rules and measurements, rather than building skills, games sense and physical literacy through purposeful and systematic education.

Instead of celebrating every child's achievement through movement and learning new skills, Primary Schools are participating in leagues that involve children who are already competing.

Why are schools competing in tennis if they don't play tennis at school? Why are secondary schools throwing people into 100m hurdle races and triple jump competitions after children have only done this twice in school?

What usually happens is that those that are 'good' (in reality early-developers or early- specialisers) are selected and the rest of the children are left to wallow in a cesspit of mediocrity and labelled as 'low-ability' or 'disengaged.'

Do you remember "Sport for All"? What a good slogan that was: there is some type of sport for all people. But select, play and adapt for the children where they are now: not trying to replicate the ultra-competitive Independent schools that use sports fixtures as an arena to showcase how much better they are than other similar school

PE can be taught well in Primary Schools.

All is not lost. Despite some poor saps being forced to complete a 'Daily Mile' (the brainchild of some bottom-feeding, business person who is cleaning up financially by exploiting imagination-starved and desperate head teachers) there are opportunities to teach our children well.

1. Realise that play and playgrounds are as important as anything being 'taught' by adults. Just look at what Greg Thompson does with hopscotch here. https://rb.gy/xryx11
(N.B. there is no point in secondary schools 'teaching' long jump if the pupils are unable to do hopscotch).

The active breaks and different markings on the ground plus certain implements like skipping ropes or hula hoops will ensure that children choose to move. When you watch how they move, you will see that not one of them chooses to walk around in a big circle for 15 minutes: so why force that upon them?

2. Teach fundamental movements and get the children to practise in an infinite variety of situations/ environments. PE is unlike the classroom: children have to move to learn, and they can not be 'educated' by sitting and listening to a teacher recite rules.
For those of you at the back of the class who haven't been paying attention, that means hopping, skipping, gliding, running, jumping, throwing, catching, braking, striking and rolling.

3. Build game sense from an early age by using plenty of collaborative and cooperative activities alongside competition. The children are great at designing their own games: many of which are inclusive, fair and interesting. Compare that with cricket or rounders: games designed to produce patient

English queuers who can stand in line and wait for 'their turn.'

If a teacher has to spend 10 minutes explaining the rules, there are too many rules. 1v1, 2v1, 2v2 and 3v3 are just about all that children under 10 years old can process. By limiting the size and complexity of the game, the teacher provides more opportunities for all the children to get involved. After a couple of years doing this and then the 10-11-year-old children are ready for bigger-sided matches. 5 or 6 a side.

I know that children do compete on bigger sides and earlier but watch what is happening closely (get off your smartphone) and you will see that only 1 or 2 in each side understand what is happening. the rest are just drifting along.

Once play, fundamental movements and game sense have been developed, the children are ready to take part in team sports such as Netball, rugby, cricket and football (if they choose them).

Summary.

Never has our Nation been more in need of a concerted effort to improve the health and well-being of our children. Instead of throwing them into the arena with 80,000 adults baying at the lions slaughtering the unfortunate victims (or 20 parents shouting at a tag rugby tournament), let us focus on outcomes of competent movers who can have a choice of activities that allow them to make friends and learn new skills and be challenged on their terms.

Those who wish to compete do so in the playground: the races and jumps and matches that are held with deadly earnestness without a pushy parent or a teacher trying to win a league table involved.

No medals or trophies are involved. Instead, the reward is a Nation of happy, active and confident children.

2: STRUCTURAL INTEGRITY: CHILDREN NEED TO DO THIS NOW

If you are thinking, "My children are too young to do strength training," then you are right.

But only if that strength training means copying an adult programme based on hypertrophy (size).

A recent editorial in the British Medical Journal (https://rb.gy/i94gw1) said this about youth strength training:

"The current approach for engaging youth in strength-building activities, sometimes referred to as resistance exercise, has been largely unsuccessful. The WHO recommends that children and adolescents ('youth') participate in strength-building activities at least 3 days per week, yet participation rates are falling below recommendations.

Secular trends in muscular strength indicate that today's youth are weaker than previous generations, and many are ill-prepared for the demands of 'rough and tumble' play and competitive sports.

Weaker children become weaker adults, and multifaceted interventions that target strength deficits early in life are needed to alter the current trajectory towards unfitness and poor health."

The good news is that just a few minutes of exercise that can be incorporated into your normal sports training session can greatly reduce the likelihood of injury.

The bad news is that children are often discouraged from participating in strength training activities.

This week, a 14-year-old girl told the deputy head teacher of a local school that she was doing weightlifting at our club.

His response?   ***"Why are you doing weightlifting?"***

Not, "Well done," or "Good for you."
Nope, he would rather disparage a young woman who is active and doing something to improve her health and fitness. I wonder why so many teenage girls stop exercising…

What is Structural Integrity?*

No one would dream of starting their house building with solar panels and roof gables before ensuring a solid foundation was in place. And yet, this happens all the time in sports.

Most of the athletes I encounter have glaring deficiencies in their structure or posture that limit their ability to progress. Loading athletes like this through volume, intensity or external weight, will lead to breakdowns.
Improving the structural integrity of the youth athlete is essential before moving on to other areas of fitness.

I help the children develop four key areas that combine to improve their Structural Integrity before progressing their training:

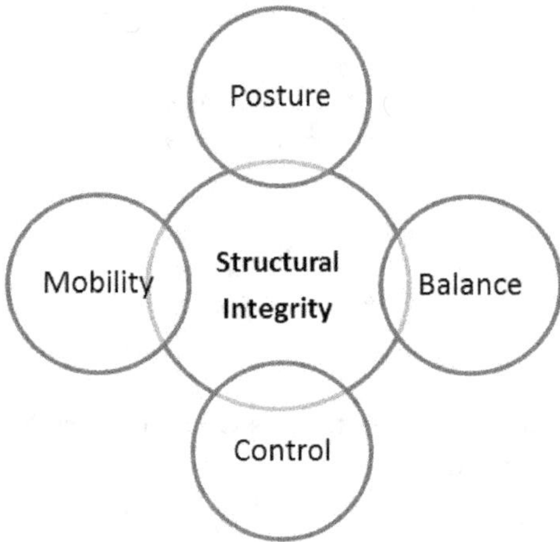

I was challenged on the use of "stability" by Dr Homayun Gharavi at a conference in Germany. He suggested that the word "control" is better than stability. Stability has been overused and is vague, the body is designed to move, unlike a table, and so control is more accurate.

What happens next?

As sprints coach Vince Anderson says, "The problem is NOT that we have athletes who have too great a spatial awareness."

Once the child can control their own body, I introduce basic exercises that can be incorporated into a warm-up or as a stand-alone session at home. From there, we expand to add movements that develop coordination, rhythm, timing and spatial awareness.

Only then do we start on our training programmes. The first month of the programme is designed to enhance structural integrity, then we add more exercises to increase the volume and intensity of the programme.

(N.B. This also applies to adults who are returning to training or starting a new fitness programme. When I do ACL rehab with professional footballers I see the same lack of structural integrity as we do in the younger athletes. The good news is that they go back to playing stronger than when they arrived).

If you think you don't have 'enough time' in your sports training sessions to work on Structural Integrity, then think about the hours/games lost through injury: can you afford for your players to be absent when you need them most?

*N.B. I thought this was an original term on my part, but then realised that it was inherited from watching too much Star Trek!

"The hull has been breached and is losing its Structural Integrity Cap'n!"

3: A NOTE ON SESSION DESIGN

A few weeks ago, I explained to a teacher my progression system for the after-school gymnastics club I coach. She was looking at the equipment layout and wondering why it had changed from the previous week.

"I either change the task they are doing, and keep the layout the same, or I keep the same task and change the layout. If I change both, the kids can get overwhelmed."

e.g. **Layout stays the same**: two mats placed in line with a bench beside them. In week one the kids roll down the mats and move back over the beams using hands and feet. In week two the kids move along the bench on their hands and feet, jump off, land and roll.

Task stays the same: In week one the kids perform a variety of jumps with shapes and turns on their individual mats. In week two they use a square space created by two adjacent mats. They move from one corner to another to learn to cover space.

"Oh," the teacher said, "that makes sense. It's so simple."

Do Simple Better.

(I took this phrase from Wade Gilbert).

Simple is underrated. If we understand what we are trying to achieve, then we can plan simple changes that will stimulate our players. If we lack understanding, we might change too much and wonder why our players get frustrated, confused or even injured.

Teachers who are given generic lesson plans, with everything detailed for them, may lack the ability to change and adapt the session according to the children's responses.

I said to the teacher, that rather than complicating the class and getting herself bamboozled (which will then trickle down to the kids), she could work on two or three themes and see how many ways she could vary those.
It might not cover the whole gamut of movement but, for someone with minimal training in that area, it would be a good start.

Can you simplify the amount you are trying to achieve and, for the next couple of weeks, vary the familiar task and/or environment for your players?

4: HOW TO STEM THE MINI-BAND EPIDEMIC

Matt, a football coach, used the phrase 'mini-band epidemic' in a message to me. I asked for clarification, he said:

"Coaches turn up with all sorts of graded resistance bands and usually stand on one leg whilst moving the other in different directions...it's become a staple in football but missing some real context."

He added:

"I also think there are better ways to use the time: we can survive without them."

If Matt means different exercises, then I might agree. If he means that no exercises should be done in football training sessions, then I disagree.

While Matt mentions mini-bands, I could insert 'Exercise X' or 'Equipment Z' and come up with a similar answer: *"Why are we doing this exercise?"*

If the coach doesn't know 'Why' then the players will go through the motions because they lack intent and don't understand what the focus of the exercise should be.

This happens at all levels of sport: a few years ago England Hockey stopped giving the men's national team players ice baths. The reason?
The German team had stopped using ice baths!

Successful coaches explain the 'Why.'

Most coaches are good at telling athletes the 'What' to do of exercises and drills, and some are good at explaining the 'How', but very few understand the 'Why.'

The social media craze of searching for quick fixes, fancy drills, and yes/no answers instead of taking the time to explain or understand may be part of this.

I produced this video (https://rb.gy/oq104h) for a rugby coach after watching her players use 'hop and hold' to warm up before a match. The warm-up was well-structured and organised with plenty of variety and progression but the execution of this exercise could be improved.

Part of the problem might be that once a club has bought equipment, they have to justify the expenditure and use it all the time whether it's relevant or not (that's a topic for another essay).

Back to the mini-bands. Why are they en vogue?

From Matt's description, it sounds like the coaches are trying to strengthen the footballers' hip muscles. Knee and hamstring injuries are prevalent in football and the min-band exercises could come under an 'injury prevention' title. Better hip control leads to better knee control at certain speeds and angles: The hamstring strain that occurs at the end of a full-speed 45-metre run to the opposition's goal line is unlikely to be prevented by these exercises.

The chances of injuries occurring when footballers land, brake, or try to turn may be reduced by improving knee control. The well-executed mini-band exercise will help strengthen the hip muscles in untrained players, leading to better knee control.

Mini-bands are also affordable, transportable and easy to use: three reasons why football coaches might like them. Footballers also feel an immediate 'burn' because the exercises target minor muscle groups: 'If it hurts, it works.'

You will notice that I am putting in a load of qualifiers rather than delivering an attention-grabbing headline like:

"Mini-bands are God's favourite exercise equipment"
(or whatever the click-bait algorithms require).

The qualifiers are there because nothing is certain: we can improve strength and hypothesise that it will reduce the chances of injury but it depends on the age/stage of the player and luck.

The chance of a single exercise being the answer to all the injury problems is minimal (despite what the Nordic hamstring researchers tell us).
Coaches need to incorporate a variety of exercises that stimulate the players' minds and bodies: even the best exercise in the world has a limited time frame before it becomes redundant or the players get bored.

Imagine eating the same food for lunch every day for the rest of your life...

We need to select exercises from a menu and incorporate them into our training sessions to give our players the best chance to succeed: either by reducing their chance of injury or improving their performance.

Sample Exercise Menu to improve knee control.

Here is an example that will help one specific aspect of fitness for footballers (and other team sport players). There may be carry-over to other aspects but the main goal is to improve knee control.

Videos for each exercise can be found in the 'Structural Integrity' playlist of my YouTube channel (Excelsior Athletic Training).
Select one exercise to incorporate into every warm-up, in addition to your normal routine (or take one of your redundant exercises out).

Hips: Hip series 1, Mini band pushback (you can see how wobbly the girls are: they need to practice more), side-lying leg lifts

Knees: Single leg squat (instead of a bench, use a football), single leg reach and balance.

Hips and knees in combination: Lunge and weep, multidirectional lunges (use a ball instead of a stick).

Good luck.

5: WHAT IS ATHLETIC DEVELOPMENT?

Long Term Athletic Development (LTAD) is a model that highlights different stages from infancy to adulthood and what types of activities are best suited at each stage.

As each human being grows up and develops in different environments, with different experiences and with different adaptations, there is no such thing as *'The ideal pathway.'* There are as many paths to the top as there are peaks.

Athletic Development is a concept that applies to all children, and for many adults who want to continue physical activity.

The ability to throw, catch, evade, slide, dodge, skip, run, jump, climb, duck, hop, roll and balance is often summarised with the term *'Physical Literacy'*.

If a child is physically illiterate, then it is unlikely, but not impossible, that they will be unable to participate in a sport successfully. They may get hurt, or injured, be unable to keep up, bend down to pick up the ball or flinch when a ball is thrown at them.

Physical Literacy can be developed through parenting.

I am often asked to provide sessions for young children- 3-year-olds in gymnastics or 6-year-olds in athletics.

If I wanted to be rich, I would organise sessions for these age groups and fill the sessions. Yet, these children do not need organised sessions at these age groups.

They need opportunities to crawl and roll on soft surfaces (sand, grass, carpets) to strengthen their limbs and discover movements themselves.

For the budding track stars, I tell the parents to treat their child like a dog. Take them down to the park and throw their child a ball, let them run around maniacally and at their pace. They will set off like a berserker and then rest for a bit. That is what dog walkers do, and with children, you don't have to pick up their mess afterwards.

But, the parent has to put down their smartphone and interact. They have to sack the iPad babysitter. The child needs the opportunity to get dirty, fall over and get up again. They need the chance to play with other children without it being a 'playdate'.

That is why I asked Willand Parish Council to improve the parks in our village eight years ago. I gave them advice on what equipment would benefit children and give them the chance to play. They have been very responsive, taking a punt on my suggestions, and have seen the popularity of the equipment since.

I was frustrated with parents not hanging around long enough for their children to play. So I suggested park benches and picnic tables to encourage families to stay. They have proven popular too, with all sorts of residents enjoying peaceful moments in the fresh air (I have yet to see any National Governing Body put in its 'Talent Pathway' plan the incorporation of benches under oak trees in parks).

Our Parish Field has become a park that people from outside our village want to visit.

Athletic Development for All.

Most things written about Athletic Development come from Sporting NGBs looking to increase medal counts or from academics promoting their model to gain speaking engagements and publication credits.

Little of what they do has any relevance to George who is 6 years old and likes playing football in the playground and climbing onto the park benches. George has no idea what a 'Talent Pathway' is.

For him, **'Long Term'** means waiting until lunchtime to go out and play.

I set up the Excelsior Athletic Development Club ten years ago. It was in response to my observations of keen young people, enthusiastic sports people, but were unable to perform simple tasks well.

Examples being:
• A 13-year-old boy who was part of a swimming 'Academy' but he did not understand how to play piggy in the middle with a bean bag.

.• Rugby 'Academy players who were given loaded back squats in a Smith machine, but were unable to stand up from a low bench without using their hands.

• Track and Field athletes who could not skip sideways.

• A 14-year-old county cricketer who could not throw overhead.

These children were given specialised activities in their sporting environment but lacked the underpinning skills and basic movement patterns to help them reach a very high level.

My work with National Governing Bodies and the Sport England "**South West Talent'** Project brought me into contact with a lot of children whose parents ferried them from organised session to organised session but had little time to play.

The so-called 'Talented' athletes were just normal children whose parents had the time or money or both to take them to training sessions.

Since I have been coaching at Excelsior ADC, I have seen first-hand how ordinary children, somewhat clumsy, sometimes tubby and lacking in confidence, can achieve a great deal given time and opportunity.

I am often contacted by parents who tell me things like,
"My daughter's got a body in a million," (can't make this stuff up) or,

"He's an extremely talented tennis player and you will be amazed by his physical ability."

I give the poor kids the benefit of the doubt and welcome them to our club session. I have yet to see any child come in and be better at the ordinary skills than our top twenty most regular attendees.

Our unsung heroes aren't county players or internationals (yet), they just come in and get on with the job of learning gymnastics, athletics, strength and coordination training, and weightlifting.

In short, they are developing as athletes. Our aim is for them to be healthy, and happy and participate in physical activity for the rest of their lives.

That is the definition of Athletic Development in my mind.

6: LONG AND STRONG: POSTURE REDEFINED

As young people go through their growth spurts, they often find a short-term detriment in skill and strength as they become accustomed to their longer levers. Their bones have lengthened but their muscles have yet to adapt.

They have become long but not strong.

Imagine rolling modelling clay out on a table. You start with a solid ball and watch as it gradually gets longer and thinner. You pick it up and it flops around: it is useful for shaping but likely to fall apart.

If a young person has grown rapidly, they have less structural integrity. We coaches need to help them adjust and adapt safely so that they continue to be active. They have become long; we need to help them get strong. This means working through a full range of motion at every opportunity.

Tension helps control

Movement is initiated by our muscles shortening, so the concept of 'lengthening' may seem contrary (Explaining to athletes as they push a stick above their head, that their triceps muscles are shortening, is a surefire way to confuse them. So I avoid that explanation). But, if we think of our bodies as moving structures, then the thought of pulling cables tight on a suspension bridge, or tightening guy ropes on a tent, then we get the idea.
(I don't use the term Biotensegrity, mainly because I am uncertain of the concept, but also because it won't help my athletes.)

Initially, most of our athletes find it hard to push a stick away from them and hold it there while doing another movement such as a lunge. As they think about the legs, the stick comes closer to their body. Slack enters the system; the body has less tension and less control. When asked to push away, they do it a bit, but when I press another stick on top of theirs and ask them to push my stick away, they find another 2cm. They have become longer (figuratively). I then remove the stick and get them to produce the same length whilst moving.

Why does this matter? Surely the lunge is a leg exercise? Yes, it is, but if we want the lunge to be a precursor to movement on the field or court, then the body has to be ready to move- the whole body.
If we are to move with control, we need tension. It is possible, and common, to do a lateral lunge by falling into it, rather than push into it. If you watch the

stationary foot of someone doing the lunge, you can often see it leave the floor, or the knee collapse in slightly. The athlete that pushes that foot hard into the floor moves fast and the whole driving leg lengthens. This same action helps with a side step.

"We want pushers, not draggers." Jim Radcliffe.

The athlete that falls into the lunge has slack in the system and will take longer to move again. Anecdotally, the draggers are more likely to get groin injuries. Getting the athlete to do a lunge whilst pushing the stick in different planes helps them learn tension and control.

A footballer needs tension in the upper body as they change direction: very often they are in contact with an opposing player fighting for the ball. They have to perform a skill with their feet, brace their upper body, lean into the other player, maintain balance and run or change direction simultaneously.
The simple lunge can be a means of getting tired or a means of getting better. I prefer the latter.

In this video (https://rb.gy/k26fhr) you can see how I transferred from the field to the gym with Frank, a centre-forward. We developed the 'long and strong' concept and applied it to lateral movement to help Frank, an accomplished athlete.

The body is a complete system, rather than a series of independent parts.

Do you remember studying series versus parallel electrical circuits at school? I spent many lunchtimes at 'Electricity Club' designing and building circuits so lightbulbs would work. Tension in our body works like a series circuit- every component has to be in place for it to work effectively.

If you want to sprint or jump, the upper body has to work in conjunction with the lower body. Slack in the upper body affects what happens to the lower body. If the free hip drops below the support hip then the support foot will be unable to recover as effectively as when the free hip is level or higher than the support hip- that can only happen with tension. When the free hip is higher, the athlete is taller (longer).

That is why you see so many running drills with athletes working with implements above their heads. It is the principle of encouraging length under tension. When you remove the implement, the athlete's body can remember the upright position and then they run faster, in principle.

Why then do some coaches and many schools insist on isolating body parts and getting young athletes to work through incomplete ranges of movement? One of our 11-year-old club members was told at his football club only to squat halfway down. Why? These poor kids spend all day sitting down, they need to move and improve their range of motion. The football coach then has them doing static hamstring stretches.

The same thing applies to machines in the school 'fitness suites': sitting or lying down removes the need for the body to have control. Our reductionist and isolationist approach to developing strength means we can do a concentration preacher curl (if that is your thing) or a leg extension, but we have encouraged slack because the external support is doing the work for us.

By squatting and lunging fully, the boy will improve his strength and length simultaneously. Pull-ups encourage length from the brachiation, so biceps junkies can get their fix and improve their posture.

None of this is new.

I regularly use exercises from Robert Kiphuth's book 'How to Be Fit' (1956 edition). I refer to them as posture exercises because, wait for it, they improve our posture.

Posture is often interpreted as a static position or series of positions. I use the term to define where our body is, its angles and how we can control it. Dwight Freeney was an incredible pass rusher in the NFL who was able to move whilst leaning at angles that seemed parallel to the turf sometimes. I would say his posture was good and he was both long and strong.

Try assuming a bad seating or standing position, the slouch. Now rectify that by moving the crown of your head towards the ceiling. You become longer and those ill-used muscles have to work.

Yoga has many different postures and poses that work on length and strength and have been developed over 1,000 years. I use some of the principles without the accompanying mystic guru baggage.

Whilst it is deemed cool to talk about 'crushing the workout', think about what crushing does to your body. It contracts and constricts your ability to move. I have a rule of thumb when asked 'How much should I lift?' – if the movement is good, they can add more weight. The moment the range of movement, or the control is inhibited, then it is time to lower the weight.

As I am training people to develop their athleticism, I can't think of anything worse than piling weight onto someone's back and talking about crushing them (unless they were doing it in a Smith machine- that is worse). A limited range of movements with heavy weights in a fixed position will help isolated muscles become bigger. But I fail to see how that transfers to movement.

By focusing on 'Long and strong' I encourage our athletes to take control of their bodies. They then maintain that control when they use external loads, or when they move faster or against opposition.

7: TEACHING CHILDREN HOW TO MOVE

It is easy to get stuck in a rut as a coach. We get comfortable with a series of exercises in our warm-ups and drills and repeat them for years on end. Occasionally we see an exercise that someone else has used and we copy it. We tend to do what we are familiar and comfortable with and ignore those exercises that are unfamiliar or that we can't do ourselves. If we limit what exercises we use with our athletes then we limit their potential.

Sports have an '*Unchangeable end-product and are bound by definite rules.*' Ruth Morison.

If we try to teach movement through sport, we are severely limiting the potential that children can achieve.

One way of removing personal bias and inertia is to use a movement framework that allows us to tweak the existing exercises. Rudolf Laban developed this in the 1950s for dance and it was subsequently adopted by physical education specialists in the UK in the 1960s and the USA in the 1970s.

I have used this framework for over ten years and am constantly amazed at how children respond.

Warning: the implementation of Laban's framework requires a set of coaching skills beyond instruction and demonstration. Coaches need to be fluent in questioning, observation, guided discovery and differentiating tasks for each level of athlete.

In the hands of trained teachers, it works well and results in a rich learning environment for the children.

Rather than taking a specific skill and reverse engineering it into linear progressions, the framework starts with each individual and allows them to discover the many ways they can move. The approach takes longer to get to a specific outcome, but it gives a broader base of movement that may allow quicker progress once additional skills are introduced.

'*Physical education students abhor the fact that they are given too much chapter and verse; taught a recognisable end-product, and not allowed more individual interpretations.*' John Foster.
Overview

Rather than constantly trying to learn and describe new exercises and dance moves, Laban designed a system that described movement. This could then be interpreted in different ways by different subjects if the instructions were general enough. This allows for exploration by the athletes. It is less good for giving a specific technical instruction to achieve a quick fix: but coaches already have that in their coaching toolbox.

The framework looks like this:

Movement Framework for Educational Gymnastics

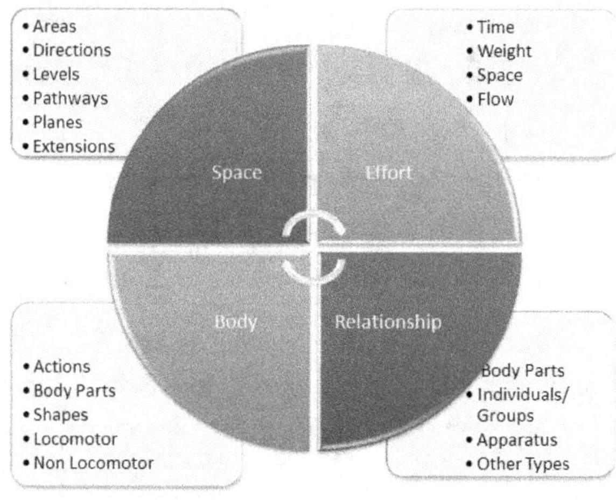

The four main aspects of movement are:

- **Body:** What is it doing?

- **Dynamics/Effort:** How is the body moving?

- **Space:** Where the movement is.

- **Relationships** (shape): How the body interacts with itself and the environment.

These aspects are then subdivided further to help refine the tasks.

For example, in Space, the use of pathways is familiar to American football coaches. But they call it something different: streaks (linear), flares (curved) and post (zig-zag) routes. Usually, the routes are very specific and confined and take time to perfect.

However, teaching these specific footwork patterns is a lot easier if the athletes have a very broad base of movement skills upon which they can build.

Under Effort, weight does not refer to an athlete's mass but the heaviness or lightness of their movement. The coach might describe running as *'lightly across the grass so that you don't damage a single blade'*. This would encourage faster leg movements at top speed.

Or, *'push hard into the ground as if you were trying to move the earth'* at the start position in a sprint race to allow more force to be expressed.

How can we use this framework?

Explaining the whole framework is beyond the scope of this article but I shall use skipping as an example.

You might already do this as part of a warm-up. You get the athletes to skip forwards for a set distance, turn around and then come back. But if you use the movement framework, then you can add a huge amount of variety to this one exercise:

· **Space:** Direction / Pathway / Levels. Skip forwards skip backwards, skip sideways in a straight line. The pathway remains the same but the direction the athletes face changes (sideways skipping is hard to coordinate). Change the pathway: instead of straight lines, do zig-zags, circles, round a box, a figure of 8, a spiral or even try to draw an elephant with your pathway.

· **Levels:** normal skipping takes place on the medium level, by trying to skip upwards or using the arms to reach up, the athletes will be moving to the upper level.

· **Body:** Rather than the standard skip action the arms and legs can do different things, that encourage and stimulate the athletes' coordination. Arms: Can make symmetrical/asymmetrical shapes, forward, sideways, upwards and downwards. Legs: can be bent/ straight, front/back.

For example, skipping with the right hand touching the left foot in front with a straight left leg and then the left hand touching the right foot behind with a bent right leg and skipping forwards, backwards and sideways before changing the sides.

· **Effort**: The athletes can do a rhythmical skip that is fast or slow. They can do an arrhythmical with a pause every 1-5 skips to show their balance and control. They can operate in a confined space to work on spatial awareness, or they can cover greater distances in a large space.

· **Relationships**: They can work in pairs collaboratively, shoulder-to-shoulder to match their partners' timing, or they can work competitively in a shadow evasion game where they try to change direction and lose their partner whilst skipping. They can go around obstacles, or over different surfaces to improve their ground contact time.

· **Combinations**: Once the athletes are familiar and competent with the different types of skipping (be patient, this is harder than it sounds) then you can combine the different movements. They can change direction and pathway whilst doing asymmetrical arm actions for example. The skipping can be combined with other movements using the framework. You can skip forwards, side shuffle sideways, run backwards on a straight pathway where your direction changes or you can keep your direction facing forwards and do the same actions where the pathway goes around three sides of a square.

Here's one I did for young children during the COVID pandemic lockdowns: https://rb.gy/umqeef

Conclusion.

This was a brief introduction. But imagine warm-ups where athletes were taken through different combinations of movement that included skipping, crawling, and running at different speeds, directions, levels and pathways. The athletes would constantly have to think and concentrate on what they were doing rather than going into auto-pilot. When the coach then came to teach specific skills, such as the wide receiver routes, the athletes would be physically and mentally ready.

Over the longer term, young athletes develop their movement competency and rarely get bored. Nor will the coach.

8: MANAGING THE TIME

If you have spent time preparing a plan for your training session, then it is worthwhile sticking to the plan. I often see coaches throwing out their plan (which must have had some thought and effort behind it) and working too long on an unforeseen problem.

Or, my pet bane as an athlete and parent, the coach runs a drill too long so that all quality dissipates and the players are in a time loop of slogging.

When I say stick to the plan, in this instance I mean, 'stick to the time frame.' Players have a certain amount of attention and concentration in their tiny little brains. Spending too much on one area risks boredom, fatigue and possibly injury.

An example session plan in rugby could be:

Warm-up: 10 minutes

Ball handling drills at speed: 10 minutes

Groundwork/ partner wrestles: 5 minutes

Rucking and mauling: 10 minutes

Lineouts/ backs moves 10 minutes

Opposed mini-games (3 different variations, 4 minutes each, 1-minute changeover).

The coach has provided enough variety to cover different aspects of the game and none are too long. But what happens in the session? The players drop all the balls in the handling drills so the coach tells them to do 'down-ups' every time they drop a ball. This reduces the speed component and makes the players tired.

The players love the wrestling work and get stuck into it: the coach loves the intensity and loses track of time, they overrun by 5 minutes. The now-fatigued players struggle with the rucking and mauling. They go through the motions and the coach keeps them going without rest (unlike a match where the ball is in hand for 1-2 minutes at a time at most).

By the time they get to the mini-games (which should be the highest intensity and replicate match conditions), there is only time for one game.

The players may be tired but the initial purpose of the session has been lost.

Flexi-time.

One thing I do when coaching gymnastics is to put a section of 'station work' in. I divide the class into two or three groups and give them different tasks: either with a coaching assistant helping them or doing self-directed tasks in pairs.

Each section lasts 5-6 minutes; long enough to get some continuity, short enough to avoid fatigue/boredom/frustration with one aspect of the class. We then have progressions/regressions for each group to allow for individual differences.

This allows us to adjust the content but keep to the timings.

However, during the initial sections, time can overrun, depending on how they respond. I am flexible on this and will adjust accordingly. I always over plan too much content so that I am never scratching my head. I have a set of 'need-to-dos' and a couple of 'nice-to-dos.'

Sometimes the gymnasts come up with a new exercise, or they are working on a specific skill, and I can incorporate that. I have this within 'flexi-time.' It is their club, after all.

9: TENETS OF SPEED DEVELOPMENT

"The hamstrings transfer force from the motor of the butt to the wheels of the foot."
Athletics coach Gary Winckler delivered an excellent overview of what he
thinks is important in speed development at GAIN.

A lot of his work is similar to what I'd seen Frans Bosch present at two
different workshops previously but Winckler has refined the somewhat
confusing Bosch ideas into some key tenets. I found his lectures enlightening
and was able to apply the lessons with our club athletes.

Training muscles for speed.

Before doing speed assistance exercises in the gym or on the track, it is
important to determine how the muscles work. There is no point doing lying
down leg curls, or Nordic curls to "Strengthen the hamstrings" if they are not
used that way in running.

The big gluteal muscles (The Big House) have a mostly parallel muscle fibre
structure and work concentrically. They are also known as *"Stupid muscles"*
because any exercise used to work them will transfer well to use in sports.

The hamstrings are a complicated bi-articular muscle with a pennate structure.
This means they are better suited to reactive forces; and not suitable for rapid
shortening.

Reactive forces: the muscles set up a system to allow tendons to do what they
are designed to do. In practice, we are looking for a very rapid transition from
a closed chain to an open chain at the moment of toe-off.

Posture is again important here: poor posture will result in either too
much deceleration due to poor foot placement, or the hamstrings unable to
utilise tendon elasticity properly due to poor pelvic placement.

The importance of the foot/ankle.

Instead of being passengers in the running cycle, the foot and ankle are key
parts of the process. Winckler uses his ears to *"Listen to it when they run."* He
can hear the ankle reactivity as there is less contact time.

As an experienced track coach, he uses awareness and sensory exercises to
help his athletes develop the right patterns. I made the point that being less
experienced, I must use drills to analyse parts of the process. I can't see what
is happening at full speed. That will come with experience.

It is important to keep a *"Neutral and active foot."* (Those athletes doing speed development work with me over the last 10 years will know about this). Winckler then took some of us through his basic drills to highlight the importance of foot reactivity.

Again, I felt better by doing something and 'Having a go.' I am unafraid to make mistakes in the hope of learning something.

I asked a question about arms, and Winckler said,

"The arms are a symptom of what is going wrong elsewhere rather than the cause." This was a good tip for me.

"Work on top speed, not just acceleration, otherwise what are you accelerating to?"

Co-ordination is the ultimate goal.

When deciding how to enhance the speed of an athlete, either in the gym or on the track, it is the coordination of the body that is most important.

This can be expressed as follows:

Strength is co-ordination training under resistance

Endurance is coordination training under prolonged or event-specific time restraints

Speed is the expression of coordination.

Strength, speed and mobility are interdependent qualities.

Weightlifting for speed development.

In the gym we did some more exercises, but this time with an external load, to enhance speed. This included hang clean variations with 1 foot behind the body, toe on the floor, then hopping up onto a step after the catch. We progressed through levels of difficulty on this drill, and this certainly challenged a few of the attendees.

Another drill was a lateral step down and up onto a higher box with the bar on our backs. The idea was to get a reactive foot action and toe up onto the higher box. This was very tricky, and Kelvin Giles got 'Stuck into me' until I had some semblance of competency.

Medicine balls.

We looked at some horizontal medicine ball work lying on your back and throwing as well as step-ups onto the step with a throw and extension at the end: this helps acceleration all the way through.

A lot of talk about abdominal work misses the point of doing it in the same environment as the sport. Winckler uses overhead bar runs, or walking with a partner doing resistive band work behind to work the hip\ abdomen area.

We also did a drill holding onto the band horizontally as it was attached to a pillar and our partner was moving it so we had to try and stabilise.

The whole session emphasised the importance of coordination (or lack of it) under load.

Summary.

Winckler was an example of a 'Sharp' coach. He is very softly spoken, but he was right on with his observations. It was great to hear some similar messages to Bosch but from a different coaching aspect.   His work in the gym was excellent.

I think we would have benefited from being on the track with Gary and seeing how he coaches hurdlers, and what he sees.

10: HOW TO MAKE YOUR TEAM FASTER

During the summer, I was asked by the coach of a local rugby team to help the players get faster. The coach said that the team lost more than they won and he thought it was down to speed.

I was happy to help. What surprised him was how little 'speed technique' I shared with the young players (15 to 16-year-olds). My rationale was that this would be lost or misinterpreted once I left. Instead, I focussed on 2 key points and coached a session that enabled the players to grasp the points and apply them.

At speed.

It sounds simple, but many teams practice at a slow speed. They often make a lot of noise and do a lot of running, but much of it is sub-maximal.

Tip 1: To get faster you have to move fast.

This starts in warm-ups: the young rugby players stood in a circle throwing one ball to each other (a common sight in rugby). One of their mums told me to leave them alone because they were 'warming up'! I ignored the mum and told the players to move after they had passed the ball.

I then gave them two other balls so that they had more opportunities to pass and catch (and they had to move more frequently). I then split them into two groups and they had to switch groups after every pass. This did get them warm.

How to apply this with your team.

Fast players stand out in football matches. The ability to outpace your opponent, with or without the ball, and to make a line break into space and receive the ball is a game-winning ability.

As with most sports, the higher the level of competition, the faster the pace of the game is: physically and mentally. It is important then to make sure that players are prepared to run fast when needed.

Whilst it is unreasonable to expect every player to be the fastest, I expect that every player can be their fastest when coached well.

Is your team getting faster or just getting tired?

To develop speed, players need to run fast, then rest and then run fast again. This seems blindingly obvious. But, working with players from three different football teams this summer, I was amazed at how little time was spent doing this. Coaches seem to want players to do 'fitness' and 'running' which involves the players being unable to stand at the end of the session. The simple principles of Progression, Overload, Specificity and Recovery were ignored or not understood.

Unfortunately, many football coaches think along the lines of, "Boxers/ Royal Marines/ Triathletes are fit, let's get one of them in to help our team.'

Examples of sessions that will not help your players get faster include:

Boxercise

Circuit training: burpees, squat thrusts, squat jumps and shuttle runs (I saw this team lose the next day: 2-0 down at half-time, they lost 11-1 (penalty) as their players gassed in the second half).

3-mile jogs at the coach's pace.

Fireman lifts and carries (led by an ex-Royal Marine where this type of activity is relevant to rescue battlefield casualties).

Footballers need endurance and the ability to play well for 90 minutes, whilst covering 8-12 km intermittently and in different directions and speeds in each match so they need to train accordingly. The sessions above got the players tired but had little to no specificity and no progression and most had minimal recovery. The players soon learn to pace themselves to be able to last the session.

Tip 2: If you want to get your players faster, they need to be fresh at the start and have adequate rest in between sets.

Build the speed up.

Running faster requires having the technical capability and the physical capacity to get to top speed. If you ask players to run 60m as fast as they can then they may find their hamstrings and quadriceps are ill-prepared. If you ask players to sprint 5m then they are less likely to get injured. They are also more likely to put in maximum effort for a short distance.
I always start coaching footballers with short sprints of 5m and 10m. I develop the distance they cover over the weeks up until they can sprint at full speed for 60m.

I emphasise the word sprint because all footballers can run 60m and many think they are running fast. But, if they are used to running 60m 'fast' and then jogging back before doing another run, then they start conserving effort and energy and run at less than top speed.

However, over 5m to 10m, they are comfortable with putting in their top effort, especially when put into partner races over short distances. I link these with physical preparation exercises and technical drills that lay the foundation for top-speed running.

So the session in week 1 might consist of:
* Warm-Up: 10 minutes.

* 5m sprints x 6

* Technical drills

* 10m sprints x 4 (2 as a race).

* Football training.

Top-speed running is a physical overload that causes the body to adapt. The hamstrings need time to adapt so I am cautious in how far they sprint. Unlike sprinters, footballers are also using their hamstrings when kicking and decelerating as well as reaching for the ball.

Flexibility work is included in the technical drills and warm-ups to help increase the range of motion and at the end of the session to help relax the muscles.

I also have to earn the footballers' trust. Once they see that when I say, "two repetitions, max speed," then that is what they do and no more, they can then stop saving themselves for whatever is next.

By week 6 the session might consist of:
* Warm-Up: 10 minutes.

* 5m sprints x 4

* Technical drills

* 20m sprints x 2

- Technical drills

- 40m sprints x2

- Technical drills

- 60m sprints with curves x 4

- Football training.

Working with the coach

None of this works if the coach is a die-hard 'flog 'em until they puke' advocate. Many coaches still run training sessions based on what they did as a player. Time is precious within the semi-professional ranks: the team needs to practice skills and tactics as well as get fit for the season. I take time to work with the coach and explain my methodology.

Two questions I find helpful to ask the coach are:

1. Do you want a faster team?

2. Do you want fewer injuries?

If the answer is 'yes' then we have a great base from which to work. I can then offer suggestions about how to improve the endurance of the team (which all football coaches are thinking about) that does not require boxercise.

11: WHAT IS PHYSICAL LITERACY?

Physical Literacy is a term gaining currency to help promote the need for children to be given the opportunities to move. Physical education has been squeezed out of the school curriculum, competitive sports have taken over and many children are disheartened and therefore disengaged.

"Partly through lack of sufficient activity, some children are awkwardly overgrown while others are fat and flabby so that eventually the desire for movement is lost and they join the ranks of the physically illiterate." Ruth Morison (1969) (1).

A physically literate individual, *"Moves with poise, economy and confidence in a wide variety of physically challenging situations."* (2).

'Physically challenging' situations could include sporting activities such as tennis, family games such as Twister, being able to play tag in the playground or copying dance moves from Ciara!

By being physically literate, the child, and then the adult, will have a much better chance of finding something they can do and like and take part in.

"If you teach them to move well, you don't have to tell them to move often." Rita Parish (3).

Literacy and numeracy are cornerstones of education in the UK and around the world. Children are educated, tested and retested continuously. There are league tables that compare class to class and school to school. There is a relentless pursuit to "improve standards".

Unfortunately, the same amount of effort is lacking when it comes to physical literacy, despite the resources having been around for years.

This video (htttps://rb.gy/xe07k0) shows me guiding my son through some ideas to help him develop his physical literacy.

Moving is learning.

"The increasing supply of ready-made entertainment and mechanical means of transport compel many children to quell their natural urge to move, and their inactivity makes them dull and passive." R. Morison

This was before iPads, and smartphones and when most families were lucky to have one car.

"Learning is the process whereby knowledge is created through the transformation of experience." (4).

If children watch TV before school, are driven to school, sit in an assembly for 45 minutes, are kept inside at break time, miss p.e. because the hall is in use for the nativity play, are driven home, watch TV, go to bed: how do they learn to move?

A worrying statistic is that in 1985 the average child played outside for 30 hours per week, in 2005 this was down to 5 hours per week (5).

That means the average 15-year-old in 2018 will have 12,250 fewer hours of accumulated free playtime compared to their 1985 counterpart.

For the 'sporty' kids today, this means they are in danger of over-specialisation and overuse injuries. For the 'non-sporty' kids this means they are lacking in basic movement skills and feel inhibited and lack the confidence to try.

Given the opportunity, children want to move and explore. In an over-mechanised society, the last thing children need is to be put on a machine to exercise. The dull repetitive nature of treadmills, adductor leg machines and cross trainers replace the joy of movement and discovery with mind-numbingly boring labour.

There is more to physical literacy than improving simple physiological functions: sitting on an exercise bike will improve your heart and lung function, but it will do nothing for balance, coordination or skill (pretty hard to pull a wheelie on one too).

"The richer the interactions, the more individuals develop their human potential." Margaret Whitehead (2001). (2).

Without these rich interactions, our children will never reach their full potential. Driving your child to a swimming lesson and watching someone else give them instructions for 20 minutes out of 30 minutes is far from being rich or interactive.

Instead, these might surprise you as examples:
Jumping in muddy puddles (kids have to be outside and in the wet, and on uneven ground).

Splashing in the bath.

Going down a slide (and climbing up the ladder to get there).

Hanging upside down holding onto parent's hands.

Wrestling with siblings.

Crawling around the house (not left in a cot or a car seat during "play dates".

Walking to school (or skipping, hopping, running, tripping, scootering, cycling, skateboarding).

Playing in the pool with family (emphasis on playing, children need to be comfortable in a strange environment before even beginning to listen to an instruction).

Hopscotch, skipping, jacks, bean bag throws, frisbee, paper aeroplanes, stone skimming and jumping over puddles are all 'rich interactions' which should be habitual before even going to an athletics club.

Throwing paper (https://rb.gy/vw88u9) is fun and will help develop the child's underlying skills.

Apart from going to the swimming pool, all the above are free and therefore should be familiar to all children. However, they require time which is precious and they may seem trivial to adults (who are often looking for the next big thing to post on Facebook).

Summary.

Unstructured, messy, disorganised PLAY, allows children to make mistakes and adapt to the environment around them. This then gives them a large database of experiences that they can draw upon when needed in the future.

If you are a sports coach or p.e. teacher moaning about the lack of movement skills in your players/ pupils, think of opportunities you can create rather than follow a fixed pattern of lessons designed 30 years ago!

If you need help or guidance on how to fix the problem, then please contact me about helping you and your team.

References.

1.   A Movement Approach to Educational Gymnastics: Ruth Morison (1969).

2.   Margaret Whitehead (2001) The Concept of Physical Literacy, European Journal of Physical Education, 6:2, 127-138.

3.   Personal communication with Rita Parish, Willand Tennis Club 2013.

4.   Experiential Learning: David Kolb (1984).

5.   Personal communication Honore Hoedt Scottish Athletics Conference 2016.

12: ARE YOU RECOVERING WELL ENOUGH?

When planning a training programme for athletes, it is easy to write down sets, reps, times, volumes, intensities and loads. Structuring the recovery programme to maximise adaptation between training sessions is harder.

With supplement companies and equipment manufacturers bombarding us with recovery aids, it is difficult to establish what is effective, and what is hype (I live in Devon: we have two coastlines and plenty of rain, yet one company has been trying to sell me 'ionised' water!)

Fatigue comes in different forms:

Central: whole body.

Peripheral: sore forearm after tennis.

Neural: Mazimal efforts such as weightlifting

Hormonal: Adrenaline rush and subsidence.

Psychological: Winning, losing, anxiety, joy.

Nutritional: Energy deficits.

The recovery process needs to target these different areas. They will all take different amounts of time to recover, and it is tough to balance enough rest for one aspect of fatigue such as physiological with another such as emotional.

For example, competing in the final of a competition may be physically easier than a training session, but the emotional, psychological and hormonal stress will be much greater and this should be taken into account.

Simple recovery tools every coach can encourage.

I use the word 'encourage' because most coaches only see their athletes for a few fleeting moments after matches (except on away games) and then the recovery is in the laps of the gods (or parents).

A note on the recovery research: much of it has been conducted in Australia and the USA, where the climate is often hot. Cold water immersion (CWI) and ice baths got a lot of attention in the early 2000s but many athletes in our climate (UK) objected to being forced to sit in an ice bath.

On a hot day, after a tiring session, I like jumping into the paddling pool in our garden. Last month, I competed in a miserably cold gym in Cardiff and the last thing I needed was more cold. I spent ten minutes in the hot shower and felt much better.

In the cold winter, my preferred (and luxury) mode of recovery would be a 10-minute pool session followed by 10 minutes in a sauna.
In the summer: swimming in the sea and lying on the beach have a similar effect.

5 simple recovery tools that are so obvious that most people don't do them!

1. Active recovery: move for 5- 10 minutes after the match (walking and talking, some stretches if you want to).

2. Drink water: at least 500ml before they get changed.

3. Eat food: a banana or a cereal bar (not a packet of crisps that have minimal nutritional value and have to be eaten with dirty fingers).

4. Praise and positive talk. If players have lost or played badly, the last thing they need is a kicking when they are down. Find something positive to say so that their minds can begin to move away from dwelling in the basement of despair.

5. Shower. (It's a thing we used to do after every school p.e. lesson and match: younger coaches can Google it). If you are travelling for more than an hour, then taking a shower is essential at the match venue. It is essential for hygiene as well as feeling better.

All of these strategies will be ineffective if your athlete fails to sleep well. All the theory in the world is redundant if they are up watching TikTok videos until dawn. If one of these 'proven' methods causes a delay in sleep, then try something else. The individual response is what matters.

Research Summary.

For those of you who want to do a bit more, here is a quick summary of how different types of physiological recovery tools compare in research:

Strategy	Pros	Cons
Passive rest	Requires minimal effort	Ineffective for quick recovery
Compression Garments	Requires minimal effort, good for travel	Expensive, requires correct fitting, inconclusive data
Contrast Water Therapy	Works well, quick,	Requires facilities, difficult for large squads.
Active Recovery	Free, easy to do, effective.	Bad weather and team talks can distract or delay.
Cold Water Immersion	Passive, effective.	Can shock the player and actually be stressful, requires facilities.

13: SPORTS SCIENCE FOR COACHES

In 2018 I had the privilege of attending a great overview of the scientific process and how things stand in this millennium by Peter Weyand at GAIN in Houston. This was better than any lecture about sports science I attended whilst studying for my MSc.

Many sports coaches either shy away from the science, leaving it to support staff or they misinterpret basic principles. Weyand, like all great coaches, explained things clearly, and methodically and I came away informed and inspired. Here are my key thoughts from his presentation.

In the last millennium, there was little or no information available to sports coaches. Peter Weyand said that much or most of what is available now is "shaky".

Here are his 5 "Drivers of Disinformation":

1. Proliferation of Information Outlets (Instagram, Facebook, YouTube, Podcasts and Twitter).
2. Volume of data and literature being produced (wearables and new technology).
3. Poor quality research training.
4. Pressure to publish (anything).
5. Self-Promotion (Not all bad, helps share ideas, but often results in self-citations).

This results in *"literature pollution"* and disinformation. Peter said that *"laziness is the default intellectual condition"*.

It is hard to filter what is good or useful in this age. In fact, *"Computers don't reduce work, they create more of it."* (Peter Taylor, 1994).

So how can busy sports coaches develop a filter and understand what will work best for their teams and athletes?

The Scientific Method.

Two years ago I was asked to present a CPD event to physiotherapists in Exeter. I gave my thoughts and observations on using motor skills learning in rehabilitation so that patients are working towards useful (and interesting) outcomes.
At the end, one physio asked *"**Yes, but what about the science?**"*

"The science"?
As if there is one all-encompassing thing, this from a person with a science-based degree showed a lack of understanding of the scientific process. Many coaches have no formal scientific background, but can still follow the scientific method.

Peter laid it out very well, and these principles will help you as a coach develop a filter.

1st: Get an idea or question.
2nd: Make observations.
3rd: Analyse observations.
4th: Idea supported: Yes/No?

Peter suggested that good researchers ask good questions and then look to first principles for answers.

Step 1: The research question must be good.
Step 2: The hypothesis must be testable. The study's design must yield data that will "get out of the noise".
Step 3: Analyse the observations in the right way. Peter used several examples to illustrate what works/ doesn't work.
Step 4: Proving and disproving: how well does data support the idea?

An interesting point was that an idea can never be proven true! Instead, the scientific method can only disprove. It only takes one outlier or piece of data to disprove a theory: the exception.

For example, Peter was studying sprinters in action and a common hypothesis was that symmetry between limbs was needed. One sprinter had a big asymmetry and yet was very fast. This one individual therefore disproved the symmetry hypothesis. Other factors must be important in sprinting.

Degrees of Uncertainty.

In the past, I have often gotten confused about what is presented as "research" compared to "theories". This is especially true in ideas like Long Term Athlete Development (LTAD), where many papers are published stating that this latest version is the definitive answer.

Peter helped me understand better the hierarchical language of degrees of certainty.

1: Hypothesis (an idea).

2: Model (LTAD is an example).
3: Mechanism.
4: Law (Gravity). Hard to argue with this.

(Peter may yet to have dealt with 'Mum Chat' or 'Bloke down the pub' which trumps all of the above! No matter what I do to try and help educate parents, they prefer to listen to their friends).

Conclusions.

This presentation helped me understand the scientific method (much more so than a whole module of "research methods" at Brunel University whilst studying for my MSc).

"If you cannot explain the conclusion in 1-2 sentences, you will never reach a general audience".

I would add that if you cannot explain the conclusion succinctly, you may be unclear yourself as to what is happening.

Peter used Isaac Newton as an example of making a big subject very simple. Newton expressed his 3 laws in simple terms and then came up with a very simple equation $F=Ma$.

When doing research (that includes looking at your own teams) it is important to ***"Get the big stuff and keep moving"*** (so much for "marginal gains"). Find out what matters most and look at that.

When reading research ***"It's critical to be critical"***.

Check the scientific method of the paper:

1: Is the idea supported Yes/ No and does it have a value?
2: Is it testable?

This will then help you decide whether to try and implement some of the ideas into your practice.

14: INTENTION AND ATTENTION

In our Freestyle Gymnastics classes, the young gymnasts spend the first ten minutes of each class working on their favourite skills. Some of them do so with a laser-like focus, repeating the same skill as often as they can, while others drift from skill to skill, using different pieces of apparatus for a few repetitions each.

I watch and interject with advice if I think I have something useful to add.

Before that, I ask, '*What are you working on?*'

Strangely, sometimes the gymnast says, '*I don't know.*'

Other times they say a skill like cartwheel, and I then ask, '*What part of the cartwheel?*'

'*I don't know.*'

The gymnast who doesn't know what skill they are working on lacks intent.

The gymnast who doesn't know what aspect of the skill they are working on lacks attention.

How coaches can help athletes get better at practice.

During the last half-term, I tried to change how the gymnasts practised in the warm-up but not what they practised (that is their choice). I explained to them that two things will help them improve their skills:

1. Intention: knowing what you are trying to do and why.

2. Attention: knowing what to think about while you are doing it.

Example: The aerial

The aerial is the common term for a no-handed cartwheel. It requires the gymnast to be able to move at speed, upside down, without hands. Many of our freestylers have the physical capability to do this but struggle to complete the whole skill.

I used this as an example to show them how they could improve their practice.

First: did they know what an aerial looks like? If not, show them a video or another gymnast doing it (there are a couple of variations).

Two: Can they think of themselves doing the skill before they attempt it? I did introduce the term visualisation here. I got them to practice this with simpler skills too.

They now have a clear intent: to perform an aerial.

Three: We then discussed what foundation moves they need to be able to perform an aerial. They came up with:

Hurdle step, speed, one-handed cartwheels (both sides), and bravery.

Four: I then challenged them on the speed, 'What makes you faster, what part of your body has to move fast?' They gave me answers such as feet, legs, hands, and arms. All of which are correct.

Five: I then asked them to think of moving one part of their body as fast as they could when they practised the preparations.

This was the attention: they were thinking of a specific body part that had to move fast.

We also did this for a couple of different preparations and practices that then led to being able to do an aerial, such as using some equipment.

How to progress and create a collaborative practice.

A couple of weeks of this, with my asking, the same questions, led to a much more focused warm-up. I then asked them to partner up and share a skill. They had to say what they were working on (intent) and what they were thinking about (attention).

This last part meant that:

a. No one got stuck in a rut, they had to practice their partner's skill.

b. They interacted and shared ideas.

c. They had to be clear in their mind before explaining it to their partner.

d. I can stand back and observe the whole scene rather than being sucked into one skill/ person.

Summary.

This method can be applied to any sport. I did this with gymnasts aged 10-14 who were comfortable working with each other. It may or may not work with younger people.

Take a skill, ask what you are trying to achieve (intent) and then what to think about to achieve it (attention).

Good luck and I hope you enjoy the benefits.

15: CREATING YOUR OWN SPORTING CULTURE

I lay out the equipment before every gymnastics session that I coach. It is mostly the usual set up but I can arrange things in a different order or shape. After I greet the young gymnasts, they have 10 minutes to warm up. This is their opportunity to practice a skill they are keen to develop or to try out new things.

In a world where they are told what to do all the time, the chance to be creative is golden. The older gymnasts have the same opportunity but tend towards working together and sharing.

This is not written down in a manual anywhere, it is something we have developed at our club. Culture develops organically and is unique to each organisation. It may even be unique to the teams/ groups within that organisation.

What works for us is a reflection of my experiences and values, combined with the help of the volunteers, and the input of our members.

I received this feedback on Monday, from an athlete I last coached 12 years ago!

"You were so incredibly supportive of me (and many other young people) in my younger years when training. You made me feel like I could achieve anything and I have never forgotten it, so thank you for helping a young woman have confidence and a belief she could achieve anything with the right mindset."
Mary.

Be genuine.

About a decade ago, a book called 'Legacy' was the darling of the coaching world. It is an account of how the New Zealand All Blacks rugby team built their culture. I saw many rugby coaches trying to inflict what they read onto their teams.

Instead of learning from the principles of a successful organisation, they tried to implement specific practices. This met with differing amounts of success and failure as well as bemused looks from 6-year-old boys and girls.

Athletes, whatever their age, can spot phoneys and will call them out (if allowed) or walk away (if unable to speak their minds).

Before you try and change the culture of your club or team, I suggest you dig deep and understand what your values and goals are. When you find that out, then creating practices and rituals becomes much easier.

A good book to help with this is, '*You win in the locker room first,*' by Jon Gordon and Mike Smith.

But what about dysfunctional culture?

"Culture (writ large) is largely built on unchallenged assumptions. Assumptions are the rust that forms in the absence of critical thought and movement." Steve Myrland.

I would suggest Myrland's quote represents 'Group-think' rather than 'Culture' per se. However, a stale culture, with autocratic or dogmatic leadership, can lead to Group-think.

Did any of you watch the documentary on ITV, last week, *"Gymnastics: a culture of abuse"*?

While you may not coach gymnastics, there are lessons to be learned from a dysfunctional culture. The reporters interviewed coaches and three victims of abuse (there are many more who are unwilling/unable/terrified to come forward) who stated that abuse of gymnasts had been normalised, especially at higher competition levels.

Having witnessed this first-hand in several different sporting 'elite' environments (and suffered from emotional abuse while competing in Karate), I vowed never to replicate this in our club.

It's why we don't participate in gymnastics competitions: they lead to a slippery slope of more training, more hours, more 'discipline' and more sacrifices (from children and parents).

British Gymnastics keep sending out surveys and glossy brochures, but they counteract this by selling competitions to 'Recreational Gymnasts.' Almost every club divides their gymnasts into Rec (bad) and Comp (Good) with the 'best' coaches coaching the Comp groups and volunteers and juniors coaching the Rec (How they think they can spot 'talent' at 5 years old is the subject of a different post!)

If we are to protect our children and create an environment in which they can flourish according to their needs and wants, then we need to challenge our assumptions.

Most children want to participate, learn and make friends. Why not allow them do that? The race to compete at too early an age is driven by parents and coaches.

Children compete in their own time and on their own terms, when allowed. Think hard before forcing them compete (especially if you are unwilling to stand on a mat alone in front of a crowd of strangers, wearing a skimpy outfit yourself).

16: HOW TO CREATE A WORLD CLASS PHYSICAL EDUCATION PROGRAMME

"If you screw up your kids, nothing else matters."
Greg Thompson, GAIN 2013.

Physical education used to be about function: getting fit to help with a full day's work and then helping with the harvest. Now it's mostly about competitive sports.

"A high-quality physical education curriculum inspires all pupils to succeed and excel in competitive sport and other physically demanding activities." U.K. national p.e. curriculum guidelines.

It doesn't have to be this way. Greg Thompson has recently retired from his role as a p.e. teacher at Farmington Schools. He presented at several GAINs and was instrumental in my learning about Rudolf Laban and Educational Gymnastics. Without him, I would be a lesser teacher.

His enthusiasm and passion are linked with a detailed knowledge of the correct physical developmental stages for children. His Games teaching is imaginative and fun, and I enjoyed being a student of his in the early morning sessions.

Here are some of the key points I took away from one of his lectures.

"Quality of design leads to user delight."
Seth Godin.

The better the design of the p.e. programme, the better the children will enjoy it.

Greg (a keen sailor) remarked that his boat has got a keel. "Unfortunately, p.e. doesn't. P.e. drifts in the direction of the latest prevailing wind. Quality content is being blown off course by marketing."

Marketing can include 'Academic studies' that use school pupils as test subjects (Personal note: often the actual intervention in a study is done by poorly trained undergraduates, rather than qualified teachers).

Moderately vigorous physical activity (MVPA) is one such wind, where heart rate is the only measure of work done. The 'dance, dance, revolution' is another. 'Fun is #1' is often the barometer of success rather than what is being achieved or giving the children physical skills for life (enough meteorological analogies now).

The one-size-fits-all approach is great for MVPA or sports-based p.e. But, the physical education specialist is an endangered species: we are on the precipice of them being replaced by $7-per-hour 'fun leaders.'

"The Moderately Vigorous Physical Activity movement has led to a generation of college professors and young teaching offspring who have lost contact with the quality movement. By pushing fun as a priority, children's "normal" has changed. They expect physical education to be game-playing. Hard work is a rarity. In our high schools, teachers fear making students in their classes perspire will lead to less students signing up for PE electives (= fewer teaching jobs)." Thompson.

The erosion of quality content leads to greatly reduced contact time and devalues the work of teachers. No one has said *"Calculus is hard, let's not bother"* so why do we do it with p.e?"

Questions you might want to ask of your child's school or your teaching:

What happens to develop physical competence?

What happens to develop skilful movement?

What happens to develop perseverance?

(Perseverance was the school motto of Merriott Primary School in 1977 when I went there).

Create an intoxicating physical education environment.

The Unicef definition of quality of teaching/education states that a good physical education teacher should be well-grounded in:

Motor Learning

Athletic Development

Social & emotional development

Inter-personal skills

If you add 'Observational skill' then you have someone who can perform 'Skilled assessment.' Does your child's PE teacher have these skills?

What about following an advanced pattern that is based on observing elite performers? An example is copying the throwing patterns of baseball pitchers for primary school kids. This is an 'error model' (see Greg's comment below).

Instead, we should ask *"Is there a known pattern of steps on the way to advanced?"* We can then set task constraints to help the child get the right outcomes, remembering that the child has a role in this process.

Physical education requires movement.

For example: throwing. A West Indian cricket fielder may run TWO steps from the boundary and sling the ball to the wicketkeeper, planting the left leg and shifting weight forward, rotating the trunk first, then the arm following through.

The key point is the lag time between trunk rotation and arm movement, so that is what the p.e. teacher should be looking at first, rather than the foot planting.

There is no point looking at a lag in the arm segments if the pupil stands face-on to the target and throws the ball underarm. Instead, the teacher might create a task constraint where the pupil has to straddle a line that is parallel to the wall, and then throw forcefully from lines that are progressively farther from the wall.

They can then progress to standing side on to the target, then to having a slightly wider foot stance.

"The idea of creating a task that elicits a positive change without having to engage in a lot of verbal instruction comes out of Esther Thelen's research on dynamic systems."

The goal of the teacher using this approach is to pick a task that lets the student 'self-organise' to the next level. So in the throwing example, a child who is not trunk rotating begins to trunk rotate when we have them straddle the line and throw hard.

We don't talk about trunk rotation with 5-year-olds, we just show them how to put one foot on each side of the line and let them back up to the next colour line when they can hit the wall from that one. The task squirts trunk rotation out.

This is a *"Dynamic systems approach to development"* (Esther Thelen).

It applies to running, skipping, sliding and jumping as well. Is your child being taught these skills?

Kids learn what they see.

So much for the theory, how does this translate into a living, breathing entity?

Greg is a great believer in using a playful approach and getting the kids to self-organise. However, before this happens they need to have a 'mind's eye picture' of what it is they are supposed to do.

Create mindfulness: the devil is in the details. Give them a why: *"This will make you a faster runner"*.

Stop the class and show them the good person. *"I like to pick someone to be my "Eagle" and spot a skilful/on-task performer. This puts the child into the role of observer."*

The environment must be right if a kid fails the task: do we give them another chance to succeed? Is it okay to make mistakes?

Try to have contact with every child in each class: constant reminders.

Kids learn what they see: we must walk the talk.

If the children are taught the individual stages according to their ability, then they all progress. This is hard work though, as anyone dealing with 29 five-year-olds can testify! Greg has got those skills and practices hard at developing them.

Compare this to the sports-based model where children are asked to remember the rules of the game: *'Only allowed to pass backwards, must run forwards.'*

Yet they are still unable to catch the ball without bringing it into chest or are unable to run without their arms crossing the mid-line of the chest. Carrying a ball whilst running inhibits that development further and they will have a forlorn hope of passing that ball accurately!

Minor rant.

Unfortunately, we are suffering from cultural amnesia as the latest generation of physical education "specialists" have graduated from a sports science background and have no inkling of what p.e. could and should look like.

They may well have been a 'Sports leader' or 'T&G ambassador' at school; they would have got a nice t-shirt or hoodie and attended lots of talks. Ask them to climb a rope, or teach kids how to run, jump, skip or throw, let alone do a forward roll and they will look at you blankly.

One 14-year-old girl at a "PE school" in Plymouth does only one hour of PE, a week. In that one hour she goes to primary schools and tells those kids that they need to do more exercise! Yet, she is unable to do a single press up or run 400 metres without stopping: what kind of madness is that?

The good news is that many willing teachers are keen to be shown skills that help them in their classes.

Yesterday I did a multi-skills club with Willand school where we looked at throwing and hopping. We based this on the rubrics developed by Greg and his team. The two teachers were excellent at spotting the stages of development and coaching the children.

It is possible to improve the quality of your physical education programme, but it requires good teachers, who have access to the correct information. More importantly, it requires vision and perseverance.

17: CORE TRAINING FOR CHILDREN

There is a tendency within the education and scientific world to measure things. We can benchmark things or test things, and then create an intervention and measure again to see if progress has been made.

Because the human body is immensely complex, we can't measure everything, so we isolate and reduce to make measurements simple. What starts as an innocent project can quickly become a dogmatic approach to training or education, where we 'Teach to the test' and lose sight of our original aim.

The plank is a perfect example of this. In itself, it is a relatively harmless bracing exercise. Very simple to teach, most people can execute it quite quickly and it requires no help. For some reason, it has become a 'go-to' exercise for p.e. teachers and some National Governing Bodies (NGBs) and then the core training is simplified to this one exercise to pass the arbitrary test.

The same benefits of having a standard test are also its downfall when it comes to children adhering to the programme (Or, in NGB speak, 'Engaging the athlete'). There is no decision-making, no discovery, no choice and no progression, except time. To get a better score, the children have to spend longer in this fixed position. At one point, the Rugby Football Union was asking its Academy players to hold the plank for 7 minutes to get a maximum score.

If I were to spend 7 minutes doing 'core training' I might spend 30 seconds in a fixed-braced position, but then I would move and do different tasks. Dr Ed Thomas told me a simple mantra for exercises that can be applied to core training,

- **Precision**

- **Progression**

- **Variety**

When working with children, I might reorder these to:

Variety

Progression

Precision.

As long as they are safe we are less worried about precision. Near enough is good enough. The variety of exercises and the progressions within them are what keep children interested.

If they are interested and challenged, they practise.

If they practise they get better.

Rather than blame the child, change the exercise.

Here are some ideas that I use, I have put arbitrary labels on them to help with ease of reading, but I use these with gymnasts, weight lifters, and sports people, from 5 years old to 60 years old.

Bracing without realising.

Once you can hold a plank or front support (press-up position) for 10 seconds, it's time to move. Children will start moaning if asked to hold one position for too long (quite rightly).

A simple sequence, but hard to execute is:

Front support

Side support

Back support

Side support

Front support

Hold each position for a count of three, then move to the next with only the hands and feet touching the floor. You can do this on forearms instead of hands to give a bigger base of support and to lower the centre of gravity.

Progression from here is 'Heel Slides' that you can see in this (https://rb.gy/anz3ar) video.

Same sequence as above, but each time move your bottom towards your heels and then return to straight legs five times. The side support movement on the one hand is very hard for taller young people who have gone through growth spurts. They curve like a banana rather than straighten like a carrot.

I use this regularly as a weight-lifting warm-up, it helps develop shoulder mobility.

The Prone Series is a staple at our club and a step up from the previous two sequences. You can see it in this (https://rb.gy/ifhpdd) video.

Partner challenges.

If children work together they make connections.

If they make connections they make friends.

If they make friends they return to training.

If they return they get better.

I find it preferable to have the children create and share tasks rather than listen to me talk.

It's a knockout (you have to be a certain age to remember this).

A task I tried this week was to have partner A in front support and partner B balance a tennis ball on the back of their hand and crawl under A without losing the ball. They then had to go over A. Partner A then attempted the same task, and then they both repeated in back support or bridge. We spent about 5 minutes on this, with much laughter, failure and talking.

Partner balance.
Partner A is in front support (knees down is the regression), and Partner B makes front support with their feet on A's shoulders. Either hold for 5 seconds then swap. Or have B walk around A on their hands maintaining the support position. Or have B roll out of the support and go into a jump or support position- making a sequence of moves.

Partner obstacle.
A is in front support (kneeling is the regression), and B puts both hands on A's shoulders and jumps over A's feet. B then crawls under A (who will have to lift their hips). Do this 5 times, then swap.

Partner lowering.
A braces himself while B stands behind and places his hands on A's shoulder blades. B then takes a step back and lowers as far as he can under control before returning A to upright. This can also be done from the front and both

sides (a lot harder). At first, the children will move about 5-10 degrees from vertical, but then they will gain confidence and strength and be able to lower to the floor.

But how do we measure progress?

All of the above tasks develop some aspect of core strength. I never time the plank as a measurement, but I do use 3 physical competency tasks I obtained from Thomas Cureton (1).

You can see them in this (htttps://rb.gy/y1c2lv) video.

1: The Frog Balance. Cureton used this as a balance test, but I think it requires strength. The centre of gravity is low and directly above the hands. Start in a squat position, put your hands on the floor close to your feet, fingers splayed. Your elbows should be touching your inner thighs. Slowly tilt forward until you feel your toes leave the floor. Hold for 20 seconds and return.

2: Side-lying leg lifts. Get into side support, arm straight, resting on the edge of your bottom foot. Lift your top leg to slightly higher than parallel and lower under control. The top score is 25, so stop then. I use this a lot because many athletes get a decent score on one side, but not the other. They immediately realise they need to improve. The other good thing is that it takes less than a minute and has a finite end.

3: Lie in the back support position and place your head on your partner's knee or the edge of a sofa. Take your hands off the floor and lift your hips until your body is in a straight line. Hold rigid for 30 seconds.

Summary.

By creating challenges and progressions I find that the children are more likely to practise than if they are just given a simple task and told to do more of it. The strength tests I have highlighted are enough for a basis.

Why do more?

We can do these at the end of a session and no one feels like they are being measured, yet they all try to do a bit better.

If I can get children to enjoy their training, work together and come up with ideas that help improve their core- strength, then I think my job as a coach is being done. Otherwise, we are in danger of just issuing pointless busy work, and no one likes that.

References.

1. Physical Fitness & Dynamic Health: Thomas K. Cureton, Jr. (1973).

18: HELPING YOUR ATHLETES DECIDE

Are your players scared or unable to make a decision in games?

Playing sports at any level requires making decisions. Sometimes they are tactical decisions such as when and where to pass the ball. Sometimes they are training decisions such as which technique to prioritise or how much weight to lift.

Players need to be allowed to make decisions to develop and succeed. The sooner they start, the sooner they can start taking responsibility and ownership, and the sooner this will translate to the field/court/arena.

Giving players choice and autonomy is one of the three key points that ensure athletes enjoy their sessions and want to return according to Wade Gilbert (the other two are learning and interacting with others).

Watching players grow and develop into independent thinkers is one of the best parts of coaching. I can't think of anything worse than standing on a sideline micro-managing every move.

But, like everything else, the players need good coaching to help them rather than leaving everything to chance.

Here are some ideas that I use to get players involved in decision-making.

Start simple.

The easiest coaching tool is exploration. e.g. before coaching a specific throwing technique, I ask the players to find as many different ways as possible to throw an implement. The safety parameter is to throw in a certain direction. I might add a restraint such as 'two-handed throws only.'

Then I get them to choose the type of throw to get the implement the furthest and practice that. In a group of 10 athletes, there might be 2-3 options chosen. I can then link the similarities to why they worked. I can also ask if that type of throw is the best for accuracy.

This can also be done with kicking and striking (racquet/bat sports).

Limit the choices.

Anyone who has done the weekly shop with a toddler will understand the benefits of having limited choices available in supermarkets, with clearly marked and labelled prices for easy comparison.

The same thing applies to sports. The athlete can choose and see which works best by creating a drill with two main options. It also forces them to work on skills that they might otherwise neglect.This is especially good for beginners who have a limited skill set.

e.g. A small-sided football game where they can only score a goal with their weaker foot or their head.

A two-handed throw either overhead standing face on, or standing side on and throwing with a long arc.

Both these examples help guide the athlete into performing basic skills that underpin good play later on but allow them to adapt to what they think works best.

Allow the athlete to create routines/games themselves.

It is important to allow athletes to take control of their training as their skill set develops and they mature. This could be within a warm-up or in the session design.

Autonomy does not mean anarchy.

It means the coach sets up situations and guides the players.
e.g. Gymnastics: create your routine that must include a balance, a roll, a jump and a movement on hands.

In invasion games: In teams of three, work out a passing move that you could do in the middle third of the pitch and then one in the attacking third. Test that against one, two and then three defenders. Did it work? Why/why not?

In Weightlifting: select a weight that you feel comfortable doing for 3 sets of 3, then 3 sets of 2. Or, here are the four exercises we are doing in the session, you select the order in which you wish to do them.

This last exercise goes against every principle of a 'numbers' coach who insists that there has to be a specific sequence to maximise results. But, allowing the athletes to choose the order themselves gives them a feeling of autonomy. It can create a 'holiday' atmosphere in a sport where repeating the same exercises is physically and emotionally hard.

Summary.

I have given a few examples of tasks that can be set up within practice to help your athletes learn to make decisions. Not all will respond, some just want to be told what to do, especially if they are tired and their brains hurt after school. Others will thrive and look forward to these parts of your training more than others.

It still requires coaching, but more of an overseeing rather than directing mode. This allows you to watch the practices and understand what is happening rather than 'doing' the practices where it is easy to lose sight of the overall session.

19: TEACHING GAMES IN PRIMARY SCHOOL

Last week, a Primary School teacher told me of her experience teaching tag rugby to year 3s (7-8-year-olds),

"We practised passing down the line a lot but, when it came to the game, they didn't know what to do."

Compare that to the advice given by the Department of Education and Science (DES):
"At about nine years of age, they may be ready to play many simple games, with three or four a side, with the object of scoring points and goals." (1972).

Have children developed a greater sense of gameplay in the last 50 years? Can they be put into competitive matches of 7+ a side because they are more skilful, athletic and tactically aware than the children of the 1970s? Is physical education being taught that much better at Primary School?

In my experience, no.

Children love playing games but they still need the time to develop. You can see in this video (https://rb.gy/xfqk9z) how these year-3/4 children are learning the basics but need help with movement.

More from the DES:
"Children at a young age play alongside each other rather than with each other."

Trying to teach pupils sport-specific skills or rules without having the foundations of game sense and skills often leads to frustration among pupils and teachers alike. Many sports clubs teach only their sport and ignore underlying movement patterns (physical literacy for want of a better phrase).

Example 1: The overhead tennis serve.
This is a highly complicated skill requiring both hands and the control of an implement, before even thinking about accuracy. Teaching this to year-one pupils is likely to result in failure.

Before attempting this skill, the pupils should be able to do two things:
1. Throw overhand properly (contralateral leg and arm, shoulder and chest rotation, elbow and wrist lag behind hip rotation).
2. Throw and catch to themselves using the non-dominant hand (for the toss-up).

By working on these two throws in the early years, amongst other skills, when it comes to time to try this complex skill, they have a chance of success. The alternative is to put the racquet and ball in their hands and let them try and work it out. This may lead to success for some who possess the underlying skill or get lucky, but many will get frustrated and stop. Especially if they only have a few attempts each due to time/ equipment shortages.

An example of doing some general ball basics can be seen in this video (https://rb.gy/vq1y34)/

Primary school p.e. is the perfect place to teach this physical literacy and that enables ALL children to learn how to move. This builds their confidence so that they can play sports if they choose or have the opportunity to do so.

What has happened to physical education teaching in the last 50 years?

Unfortunately, the dismantling of the teacher training syllabus that now leaves them with 4 hours of Physical Education training, has created a wasteland of well-meaning teachers who lack confidence and knowledge. This has opened the door for outsourcing to sports coaches who try to teach their sport to children at too early an age.

National Governing Bodies (NGBs) are desperate to 'increase participation,' and have the resources to offer beleaguered Head Teachers looking for a solution to a problem they do not understand.

Children queue up to learn rules and terminology rather than move, learn, and have fun. The teachers are given colourful 'flash cards' and 'resources' that they can read from.

But, if they don't understand the premise behind physical education, then the chances of children learning are haphazard: a few will get better, some will get better DESPITE the lesson, a few will misbehave and most will come away a bit tired (optimistically) and have learned nothing.

Each NGB is fighting for a piece of the pie so they try and recruit early to get ahead of the other sports. The poor children (and parents) are then caught in the race to specialise early. This is problematic for two main reasons:
There is zero evidence that specialising early leads to success at an adult age.

By focussing on sports rules, only the early developers and those with exposure elsewhere 'succeed.' Everyone else gets disheartened, bored or finds something else to do.

How sad is it to hear children say, 'I'm no good at sport,' at 8 years old?

They shouldn't be good/bad, they should enjoy playing games. And that's where Educational Games come into play.

Helping Children Develop Their Games Sense.

Premise: skill development and decision-making for game players are interlinked and should be taught together.

By using a framework to operate from, teachers can plan lessons easily and allow pupils to be more involved, and creative and learn at their own pace. Playing specific games requires the learning of often complicated rules that require the child to memorise as well as trying to control their own body, control an implement and deal with opposing team members.

Developing the children through Educational Games means that they are then able to learn sport-specific skills and apply the rules more easily if they choose to participate.

Outline:
Below is the framework for teachers to use to plan their lessons. Each workshop I run draws on different aspects of this framework to show how it can be used in daily teaching.

I teach different lessons depending on the age/ stage of the children and explain which aspect I aim to develop in each lesson.
The aim is for the teachers to see the overall strategy, see how it is implemented in a single lesson and understand how to develop the children from there.

Framework for content selection.

PURPOSE

Personal Meaning + Significance

POSSIBLE RELATIONSHIP
A: Specific Game
B: Combination of more than one game
C: Combination of Elements in Many Games

Game Play Development

MOVEMENT CONTENT
Nine Themes

MANIPULATIVE ACTIVITIES
Striking, Throwing, Catching, Collecting, Propelling, Carrying & Dodging

OBJECTS
Balls, Bean Bags, Rings, Pucks, Shuttlecocks, Frisbees.

IMPLEMENTS
Racquets/Paddles, Bats, Sticks, Scoops,

EQUIPMENT
Posts/ Nets, Markers/ Bases, Cages, Targets, Rebound Surfaces, Tape, Tees, Rope

Movement underpins every sport

Every lesson has some movement aspect in it: the children can not be too physically literate. There are nine themes that I use (based on Laban's work) and they can be integrated into every lesson.

Instead of a series of drills that have to be memorised, the children get to develop their own patterns through some guided discovery, exploration and solving of tasks. This requires less demonstration/correction from the Primary School teachers (much to their relief).

One of the reasons that children struggle with physical literacy and games sense is that the teachers lack the confidence to teach them. Every teacher can read and write, not every teacher can throw, catch, skip, run, jump and strike a ball.

Nine Movement Themes for Organising and Developing Educational Games Content

1. **Awareness of the Body** (with emphasis on general locomotion and the use of body parts).

2. **Awareness of Space** (with emphasis on general, personal, directions and extensions).

3. **Awareness of Weight and Time** (with emphasis on using different amounts of force and speed).

4. **Awareness of the Flow of Movement** (with emphasis on the integration of Themes 1,2 and 3).

5. **Awareness of Simple Relationships** (cooperative in nature).

6. **Awareness of the Body** (with emphasis on specific locomotor and no-locomotor patterns).

7. **Awareness of Space** (with emphasis on pathways and levels).

8. **Awareness of Time, Weight, and Space Combinations** (with emphasis on effective and efficient movement).

9. **Awareness of Complex Relationships** (cooperative and competitive in nature).

It is very rewarding to coach children and see them develop. It is almost as rewarding coaching teachers and seeing them grow in confidence as they realise there is more to physical education than rules, queues and shooing chickens.

20: A MILLION SPORTY GIRLS QUIT SPORT

A report by 'Women in Sport' found that a million teenage girls in the UK had recently dropped out of all sports despite considering themselves 'sporty' at Primary School.

Girls were less likely to do non-school club activities or 'keep fit' by themselves than boys. Two of the main reasons (and there were many, varied reasons) for dropping out were:

1. Being 'judged'.
2. The sport was too competitive.

Whilst some parents are thrilled about their four-year-old winning a medal, they might not be thrilled when that girl drops out of sport at 14 because of the pressure. But most parents, understandably, only think about the immediate future of their child.

One way of judging if your child is 'doing ok' is to see if they win medals or collect certificates. These are short-term methods of motivation (known as extrinsic rewards) that do not build for long-term participation and activity.

This is unsurprising. Nine years ago, I set up my sports club to offer a place where young people can learn new skills, play and make friends. I did this after seeing the broken bodies and tormented souls strewn across the wasteland of 'elite' sport.

Winning and performing come at a cost. I wanted to offer local children the chance to be coached well, without the pressure of competition and being judged. We offer gymnastics, athletics and weightlifting for people aged 6-43.

Over the last seven years, only three gymnasts have asked to compete. The rest are happy to participate and show their skills in an end-of-term display. When I shared the results of the survey with our club members, one mum, responded,

"Boom! Love this -one of my (many) soap box rants is adults ruining the fun for the kids in sport."

Adults ruining the fun for the kids in sports: that includes teachers, coaches and parents.

Fun is not a swear word.

The idea of 'having fun' is sometimes dismissed as puerile or childish. Yet, teenagers are still children rather than mini-adults (who thinks adults have too much fun?) and need to be allowed to create their sense of purpose and identity rather than have it imposed upon them.

Having fun does not mean trying to create a circus and the coach acts like a clown. It means creating an environment where children can develop and improve and solve puzzles and challenges appropriate to their age and stage.

Dr Wade Gilbert has identified three things that athletes like in their sessions to satisfy their basic needs:

1. **To learn and feel competent** (Am I improving? Can I do basic skills?).

2. **Choice and autonomy** (I just want to be left alone for a bit. I want to work on my cartwheels).

3. **Feel connected to others** (I like chatting. I can play with my friends. We can share ideas).

Winning is not everything: it's not even mentioned in these basic needs. Coaches and teachers who can create an environment that matches the needs of the children, rather than the needs of a sport that is looking for 'talent', will be rewarded with committed and happy members.

Empowering girls.

Another mum wrote to me:
"Thanks for the newsletter, James. My thoughts echo yours regarding; girls and sport. I also like the fact the gym kit is comfortable, unisex and therefore empowering for them!
Your point about competitions rings true with my niece. A tiny six-year-old girl who had to spend hours on a Saturday at a competitive event.
She got hungry and stressed but won all her entries, only to dissolve into tears on the podium when presented with a silly amount of medals. The pressure got too much and nearly put her off for life!"

Imagine loving gymnastics so much but an adult-led event puts you off for life.

Empowering girls can be done with a few simple steps:

1. Never assume that knowledge and skills are stable or have been previously learned. Start simple and add progressions for those who can and regressions for those who are struggling, or need more time. Here is an example using

handstand progressions (https://rb.gy/hi7c7q).

Every child starts at the beginning and as we progress they can stay on the previous level if they wish. This is still practice and they are confident they are doing something constructive. Going through the progressions acts as revision and fitness for those who can do the handstands.

2. The perception of choice is as important as choice. By allowing the children to choose whether they move on or stay on a level, they get to do what they feel is right. We also give options within a framework of movement such as jumping. Here, I set up the task and Jack can choose how to solve the problem (https://rb.gy/hiufnw)

It's a choice within a framework of learning.

We also allow free choice for every child at every session to work on the skills that they want to do. It's their club, after all. A ten-minute period where they can explore and rehearse. It is rare to see a child sit still or do nothing in this period.

3. Finally, when new members come to the club, I introduce them to another member of a similar age or the whole group in the smaller sessions. We then do partner warm-up exercises such as throwing and catching or strength exercises that require collaboration rather than cooperation. Here is an example: (https://rb.gy/vzh0yx).

This enforced social interaction is done to remove my voice from the tasks and get the children used to working with others.

At some point in the lesson, we can then do partner drills or routines so they get a chance to chat and interact. I learned a long time ago, when coaching athletics drills, to warm up by doing a concentrated drill for up to 40 metres and then allow a walk back and chat. The girls were going to chat anyway, I'd rather they do it in the rest period, than when I was coaching or they were doing it!

Summary.

If we want teenage girls to continue to exercise and participate in sports, then we need to realise that we have to adjust our sessions to meet their needs. That doesn't mean using fads, technology or gimmicks, it means using sound coaching and teaching principles that allow the girls to fulfil their basic needs.

That way, we hope that they become healthy, active and happy adults.

21: COACHING WITH COMPASSION OR FOR COMPLIANCE

"Effective leaders bring out the best in people, they do this through inspiring hope, being mindful and coaching with compassion."
Richard Boyatzis.

Boyatzis led the 6-week course I did a few years ago called, "Inspiring Leadership Through Emotional Intelligence".

The premise of the course was to make students more aware of our emotional states and how it impacts our decision-making and interactions with others.

It showed ways of creating true empathy which genuinely opens up to the other person which is very powerful (the less effective empathy is seeing the other person through a reflection of yourself.)

It showed how inspiring hope and dreams are important coaching tools. Athletes respond to that and sometimes get caught up in what other people think they 'ought to do' rather than what they 'love to do.'

It showed how being mindful is important for my relationship with athletes (I can respond better to their needs and desires) and also for my benefit (clarity of thought, renewal).

It was tough, with a bigger workload than expected, but well worth it.

"When we use the term compassion, we go beyond the typical Western interpretation to one coming from Confucian philosophy. Compassion is the experience of benevolence, of being open to others. It is caring for others who might be in pain (more hedonic), those in joy (more eudemonic) or those in search of growth (eudemonic)."
Richard Boyatzis.

Who has inspired you?

Try this simple exercise: take 5 minutes out and write down a list of people who have inspired you throughout your life. It could include family, teachers, coaches, colleagues and friends.

Think about what was it they did that inspired you. Remember as much detail as possible, again write it down.

If you have done the exercise, well done. How did you feel when you were doing it? Probably pretty good.

You have activated the parasympathetic nervous system by thinking of positive emotional attractors. You are now in an open state of mind and have experienced some 'Renewal.'

Our daily lives are filled with encounters and events that are quite stressful: being held on the phone, dealing with the National Governing Body that wants meaningless reports, being stuck in traffic etc..

This activates the Sympathetic nervous system which is good when you need to focus on an essential task or deal with an immediate event. The downside is that it limits access to all of your neural networks and the excess cortisol produced hinders your immune system.

You become narrow-minded and risk illness.

A daily dose of Renewal helps counter this: play, moderate exercise and learning new things are examples of how to activate your Parasympathetic system.

One of the discussion points in the course was:
"What ratio do we need to have between the Positive Emotional Attractors (PEA) and the Negative Emotional Attractors (NEA)?"

We need to consciously build in PEA time due to the amount of NEA we experience. For me, it was about 5:5 normally and 8:2 if I was thriving.

Hearts, Minds & Bodies.

As a coach do you activate the PEA in your athletes or the NEA?

I have found myself in the past looking to 'fix weaknesses' in athletes.
By focussing on their 'problems' it means that I am less tuned into them as people.

I now try to win their hearts by inspiring hope, explaining why we do what we do, and getting their bodies to follow.

Some coaches are very good at this and create an environment where ***'eyes are shiny with the art of possibility.'***

If you think of how NGBs often try to get their athletes to get fit, you will see how flawed it is. They put athletes through a series of fitness tests and then tell the athletes what they are bad at (NEA).

They give out a bit of paper with some exercises with funny names. Give a quick demonstration (often by sports coaches who are poor at them) and say 'Do these at home' (compliance).

They see the athletes again in 6 weeks and tell them off for failing to do their homework! 'They are not engaged.'

They test the body, confuse the mind, and then break the heart! (This is why I refuse to work in that type of environment and have resigned from some contracts).

The key to sustaining good effective coaching is building relationships. One way to do that is to focus on what people love to do rather than need to do. Find out what the athlete is good at and build from there. Once trust is established, a shared vision can be created that is very strong and will lead to success.

Summary.

I learnt huge amounts in this course. It enabled me to deepen my relationship with a lot of the athletes and coaches I work with. That has had immediate results in their performance which was unexpected.
I have also ditched some work that was just too negative. Life is too short to be dragged down by trolls!

22: THREE DIMENSIONAL AGILITY

Agility training is often perceived to be conducted on two feet. Whether programmed, random, game or task-orientated, it usually consists of a change of direction on a left–right and forward–backwards continuum.

Yet movement rarely takes place in just two dimensions: subtle and not-so-subtle changes of height and depth also take place. A boxer bobbing and weaving or a gymnast doing a double front somersault both have to move their centre of gravity up and down as well as sideways and forwards respectively.

I have found many sports coaches reluctant/ hesitant to get up and down in training despite their players doing it in the game. Here are some ideas to help you build it into your training sessions.

Levels and Pathways.

In Chapter 7, I described Rudolf Laban's framework and how it can be adapted to sport. The use of pathways, whether they are linear, curved or zig-zagged, occurs in every sport. The wide receiver route tree in American Football is a clear example of this. It contains multiple pathways such as streaks (linear), flares (curved) and post (zig-zag) routes.

The changing of levels (high, medium and low) also occurs in almost every sport. The definitions are:

High Level: Movements that occur above the shoulder height.

Medium Level: Movements that occur between shoulder and hip height.

Low (deep) Level: Movements that occur below hip height.

For example, volleyball players dive for a dig (low), block at the net (high) and move around the court (medium). (N.B. All footwork and gait occurs on or near the ground but the torso is not displaced significantly so walking, skipping and running are all described as operating on the medium level).

Coaches are adept at identifying the two-dimensional movement patterns in sports and replicating this in training drills. The coach also writes down their plan in a two-dimensional format: using either a pen and paper or a tablet.

What coaches may neglect is the changing of levels within one movement sequence. For example, Mixed Martial Arts Training (MMA) can sometimes be planned according to 'Stand-Up' and 'Groundwork'. Fighters train both on their feet and on the ground. Yet a key part of the fight is the transition from one to the other, and perhaps back again. The fighter goes from medium level to low level, their feet move along one pathway, whilst their upper body and head may lead or follow a different path. This must be done with feints and avoiding getting hit because the opponent is rarely stationary.

The rugby union lineout results in a high-level catch but it is preceded by a coordinated movement on the medium level with at least two other teammates. What used to be a straight-out up-down jumping competition between two opponents has now become a complex movement pattern involving feints, misdirections and curved and linear pathways at the medium level.

The ability to get up on your feet and back into the game quickly is another important part of playing rugby. Rugby coaches are adept at teaching tackle technique to make it more effective but what happens after the tackle? I would suggest that forwards need to be agile in the line out and from the floor and their training should reflect that.

This video (https://rb.gy/jdz1ql) shows some ideas.

Sometimes the transition between levels is more rapid such as the dive for a ball in cricket and a return to the medium level before throwing. Goalkeepers in all sports have to work between the levels and transition smoothly between them. Coaches with this position group may be the most aware of the need to plan up and down as well as side to side.

Coaching the transitions.

Once you have identified the different levels that operate within your sport then you can start to plan how to train at those levels and switch smoothly between them.

A player's body management that involves:
• rising/falling
• rolling
• jumping and landing
should not be assumed. Instead, it should be coached and developed.

One of the simplest ways to develop body management is to get your players moving at the low level at some point in training instead of the medium level. This figure-of-8 drill (https://rb.gy/tqgg1q) is one of a series that I used to help the football goalkeeper become more comfortable and resilient with working on the floor:

The loading of the hands, wrists and shoulders contains a conditioning element too. I would suggest starting short and simple and then building up.

Returning to cricket, fielding throwing and catching progressions using games are commonplace but the coaching of side rolls is uncommon. Cricket outfields are hard and players can get hurt if they dive outstretched without being able to roll and dissipate the impact safely.

The ability to catch at low levels requires mobility and practice and can be developed in the warm-ups as shown below:

1. Two hands: medium level (ball between hip and shoulder) in place.
2. 5 Lateral lunges on each side then catch medium level with side step (ball thrown to receiver's side).
3. Catch low level (below hips) in place- squat to catch.
4. 5 side rolls each side then catch low level (ball thrown to side and low for the receiver) with a dive and roll.
5. Catch high level (above head) in place.
6. 5 vertical jumps then catch higher balls.
7. Random throw and catch games using all 3 levels and both sides.

Alongside 'sets/reps'-type progressions I use apparatus to encourage (or force) players to adapt and move at different levels. A skipping rope is cheap and easy to obtain. If one player holds an end high, and another low, the other player(s) can progress up/down the rope moving side to side using whatever agility method you like.

Boxers can weave side to side and hockey players can dribble the ball around cones. The constraint of the rope height allows them to get used to that gradual transition from high to low. This saves a lot of coaching breath when working with hockey players who like to bend from the waist rather than sink their hips to a low level and look upright.

Conclusion.

Agility is fluid and dynamic and often requires subtle variations in height as well as the big 'steps' or 'cuts' that leave a defender grasping air. By getting players more comfortable at working at low levels the coach can then work on transitions between levels. Players who can do this effectively and efficiently are less likely to get injured and are more useful to the team as they are 'out of action' for less time.

23: MOVEMENT IS THE FOUNDATION OF SPORTS INJURY REHABILITATION

Dr Grace Golden gave an insightful presentation on returning to sporting activity at GAIN 2018. I liked her systematic approach which was well illustrated with video examples. She uses a large amount of creativity and fun in her rehabilitation sessions.

Grace is a proponent of Rudolf Laban's movement framework. Her ideas have helped shape how I help rehabilitate injured athletes as well as improve my coaching. I'm privileged to know her.

Coaching the injured athlete.

Grace coaches the rehab sessions, which is different from the experiences of many athletes who are returning from injury. Grace understands the need for skill development and fun in the rehab process. She often works on the sidelines with teams and integrates the rehab with the sport training. This is very important for athlete morale (it also helps remind the coach that the athlete is still alive and kicking).

Communicating between members of staff is also important. The rehabilitation world uses inconsistent language when working with injured athletes:

Return to activity.

Return to sport.

Return to play.

Return to competition.

What are we trying to do? All of the above are different in intensity, but athletes are often told to, "*Rest for four weeks,*" by a medical professional. There is a difference between graded exercise progressions and competing in a regional tournament.

Tenet 1: Start simply.

Practise and evaluate locomotor skills in isolation. This means training in single planes and one direction of movement at the start. Work on the fundamentals before athlete-specific and specialised movements.

'Criterion-based rehab,' may be a better method than, *'Timeline-based rehab.'* Grace uses the single-leg squat (SLS) as one criterion. One target is to do 70 sets in 2 minutes, ideally with a 90-degree knee angle, but 70-90 degrees is acceptable. The athlete rests for 2 minutes then repeats, building up to 3 sets total.

This prepares the athlete for 2 minutes of running or jogging better than "rest". Having objective criteria improves understanding between athletes, medical staff and coaches.

Can your athletes do 70 single-leg squats in 2 minutes when healthy? Are they fit to play now?

Tenet 2: Common agility tests should not serve as the primary training stimulus or pathway to progression.

Whilst agility tests like the Illinois agility test, the 3 cone test, or the T-test may have a place in training, they are very simplistic. This means they are quickly learned and the stimulus is redundant after a few attempts.

Better to think of a variety of exercises using different stimuli. This includes decision-making in a controlled fashion.

Tenet 3: The order we combine locomotor skills influences acceleration or deceleration exposure.

The injured body part is loaded more in deceleration activities than acceleration, Grace trains acceleration early or first and then adds deceleration.

(See Damaging nature of decelerations).

Tenet 4: Add discrete skills in transitions for directional and plane changes.

(As long as they have been trained previously). Grace broke this into 4 different phases:

Continuous direction and continuous speed.

Continuous direction and multiple planes.

Multiple directions and multiple planes.

Multiple directions and continuous planes (cutting progressions).

Tenet 5: Be mindful of how what you are doing today is preparing the athlete for what they need later.

Or, '*Start with the end in mind.*' The goal of rehabilitating injured sportspeople is very different from rehabilitating the normal population. Jogging on a treadmill pain-free could be a successful outcome for Joe Public. That is nowhere near enough for a field/court team sportsperson, so the rehab process needs to be structured along different lines.

Summary.

I have barely touched the surface of Grace's presentation on sports injury rehabilitation. Her presentation was rich with detailed examples of the exercises she uses. Most important for me was how she integrated the work with the coaching staff. It is all too easy to rehabilitate in a clinic room that doubles as a bunker.

24: REDUCING FOOTBALL HAMSTRING INJURIES

Hamstring injuries account for approximately 17% of all injuries in soccer. They mainly occur during change of direction movements, when accelerating to top speed and when overstretched. They are more likely to occur at the end of each half when the players are fatigued.

I coach several professional soccer players in the UK. To reduce the chance of them suffering from hamstring injuries I use three main training methods:

1: **Moving in different planes at different speeds when warming up** (preparing for a change of direction).

2. **Running at top speed:** the hamstrings work differently in sprinting than jogging and fast running. Hamstring injuries rarely occur when jogging.

3. **Hinging exercises in the gym:** the hamstrings cover both the knee and hip joints and exercises in the gym that replicate a hinge action help strengthen them.

You can see an example of this with one player that I coached in this video (https://rb.gy/ysadaw).

There are three hamstring muscles and they all work slightly differently. No single exercise will strengthen or prepare all three muscles for their different roles in a soccer match. I use a variety of exercises that challenge the hamstrings in training to prepare them for the rigours of the soccer match.

1: The warm-up.

I use multi-directional lunges with different arm movements to strengthen and lengthen the hamstring and groin muscles before we start any sprinting drills. The hamstrings help control the knee during a change of direction.

Adding different reaching and leaning movements to the lunges increases the difficulty of the balance and braking action in the lunge. The hamstrings have to work harder and smarter to prevent the player from falling over or wobbling. As the player becomes more competent, the speed of movement can increase and more complex patterns linked together. We spend 2-3 minutes doing this before anything else.

Here are two examples: https://rb.gy/0onugm and https://rb.gy/wfm5j3

2. Top-speed running.

The hamstrings are likely to get injured when fatigued and when used at top speed. Therefore we need to run slightly longer and faster than what usually occurs in a match.

If we just look at average speeds and average distances and train for those then the body is unprepared for the outlying top-speed runs that happen once or twice in a match: and that is when the hamstrings will be taxed most.

I include one or two 60-metre maximal speed efforts every week during the season but only after the players have prepared in the preseason by gradually increasing the sprint distance. They are unaccustomed to longer recovery periods so we do some light ball skills for 2-3 minutes in between the runs. As one player said to me when we moved from 50m -60m sprints,

"My legs definitely felt like they were in alien territory."

Time must be taken and a clear explanation given to the players so that they understand the need for max speed and max recovery. They are very good at doing repeated runs with minimal rest to improve their fitness and will try to shorten the recovery!

Top-speed running is not something where *'If one is good, ten must be better.'*

Care must be taken to only run fast when warm and fresh, not the morning after an evening match in case the hamstrings are still fatigued.

3. Hinging exercises in the gym.

These can be done with dumbbells, medicine balls or barbells. This is not a maximal strength exercise. Instead, lighter weights moving faster and with control are more suitable for the soccer player. If you do too much strength work with too heavy a load, then you risk fatiguing the hamstrings to the point where they can not cope with playing soccer.

Remember that our objective is to help the player perform on the pitch rather than win a competition in the gym.

The progressions I use are:

1. Unloaded hip hinge against the wall: get the players to feel like they are shutting a car door with their backsides. The wall gives them an endpoint for the exercise. The knees should be slightly bent.

2. Single leg hip hinge, as above but with one foot placed on the wall. This is difficult.

3. Two-legged hip hinge with a small load: medicine ball, dumbbells (held with straight arms that stay close to the legs) and maybe a light barbell.

4. One-legged- as above (video here: https://rb.gy/hbywsz)

5. Free-standing single-leg hip hinge with the free leg moving from rear to front as the hip hinges (shown in the highlight video). Unloaded to start or with a broomstick and then add a small load. This exercise requires good balance and control where the emphasis is on the speed of movement rather than how much weight can be lifted.

Summary.

These are the three principles that I have used over the last 10 years, modifying according to the age and stage of the player. At all times, I am conscious of balancing what I do with the work that the player does on the pitch.

Too much hamstring training can lead to injury as well as too little. *'Little and often'* is the best mantra for the players that I have found.

25: SPRINT TRAINING FOR CHILDREN EXERCISE AS MEDICINE

The idiom, **'Sprinters are born, marathoners are made,'** assumes that genetics is the major factor in sprinting. That is accurate if your goal is to become a world-class sprinter.

However, if you are an average human being and your goal is to run faster, then environment and coaching become important factors too. This is especially important with children.

The modern-day child is less active and has less 'free play' than those of yesteryear. Imposing a technical speed training system upon them is likely to fail: they lack the physical and cognitive capabilities to cope.

By observing how children play, and using my technical knowledge of what good sprinting looks like, I try to create training sessions that are fun and purposeful. The ideas may be of use to those of you who coach children and also those who coach adults in different sports who have not got a 'sprint' background.

The raw material needs to be shaped.

In one of the many false dichotomies thrown up in coaching, there seems to be a conflict between a free-play, laissez-faire approach, and technical coaching.

'Natural talent comes through,' or

'My technical model is better than everyone else's, so athletes need to follow that.'

To address the first point, children need to learn to run fast, it doesn't just happen. 'Learn' does not mean being 'taught' by a coach: the learning can be implicit. But, in many societies, this implicit learning does not happen because the children have limited play time (Jamaica seems to be an exception).

A study in the Netherlands looked at children's activity outside, from 1985-2005. They found that in 1985 the average child played outside for 30 hours per week, but in 2005 that had dropped to only 5 hours per week.
This has a huge effect over time:
• 1 week = 5 instead of 30 hours a week
• 1 year = 250 instead of 1500 hours a year

- 10 years = 2500 instead of 15,000 hours in 10 Years.

So, when a 15-year-old girl walks into an athletics club, the 2005 version would have played outside for 12,250 less than her 1985 counterpart.
(Personal Communication with study author Honore Hoedt. Scottish Athletics Conference (2016).

Imagine how our COVID lockdown children will have been affected.

During those additional 12,250 hours of outdoor play, the girl will have walked, skipped, chased, escaped, dodged, fallen over and been out of breath. She will have learned balance, coordination, reaction and racing without adult involvement. The raw material has been moulded and developed. In this environment, the children will know who is the fastest and the 'natural' sprinters will rise to the top.

Compare this to the 2005 child, or the 2021 child, whose parent keeps them inside except for their twice-weekly visit to an athletics club where they can be taught how to run.

The head of PE at my daughter's secondary school said to me last month, *"You wouldn't believe how many of the recent year 7 cohort run with their arms stretched out behind their backs Fortnite style!"*

Key point: the modern child is less ready to receive formal coaching than previous generations. We need to recognise and adapt how and what we coach.

Games with purpose.

As I waited in the school playground for my children to go into school I watched how they played: brief, intermittent bursts of activity, followed by some walking or standing and then more bursts of activity.

When the school gates opened and the children ran into the park the same thing occurred: this time using the playground equipment and maybe a dog or two. Nowhere did I see queues of children lining up to move one at a time and then told what to do by an adult.

When I first visited an athletics club to 'learn' about speed training, I saw a lot of standing and waiting and then a brief spell of activity before returning to the back of the queue.

I learned a lot about queuing but very little about sprinting.

I decided to structure my sessions according to how children organise themselves. I shape the activities to elicit an outcome or response that fits into the overall strategy of 'running faster.' Some parts of my sessions are not specific to speed but help the sessions flow or get the children involved early.

If the children feel like they are making progress, they are learning something and they get to share and collaborate with their friends, then they are likely to return the following week. If they keep returning they get faster.

The Framework.

Here is an example of a sequence that I follow. The drills are less important than why/when I do them.

Warm Up 10 mins: get moving, wake up, shake off the school shackles.

Either: A restricted area game of tag/ follow my leader
or: Play on the equipment parkour-style
or: Coordination challenges with balls and objects such as juggling or pass/ move.

Fundamentals 10 mins: Speed-related activities.

We keep the same ideas but change the directions and orders that we do things.
Skipping: forward, backwards, sideways. With/without arms. In lines or a square with a change of direction at each corner.
Change of movements either on command, at a cone or following a matching partner: walk-skip, skip-run, run-skip, hop to skip, walk to skip and so on. 5-10m for each.
Foot taps (ankling) on the spot/ moving forward. 'Happy feet.'
Hip locks: stationary to walking, singles to doubles. Using sticks/ ropes/ bands. 'Push to the sky and pause.'
The hip locks are the most technical that we get with the younger children and they are put in once the children are warm and receptive.

The theme of the day for 20 minutes: Drills to work on one aspect of speed.

This will include a competitive element while we work on starts, acceleration, repeat speed, reactive speed, or top speed.

I always handicap any competitive element: I select the pairs to match them evenly or if they select, I give one a head start. The idea is to get each child racing as fast as they can, regularly. If I have done it correctly, there is a close finish each time. The pairs are working concurrently for some of the session and consecutively for the remainder.

I don't want the fast children becoming complacent and I don't want the slow children becoming disheartened. I swap the partners as necessary to avoid potential conflicts. The fast children need to learn how to lose and the slower children need to feel what it is like to win. I aim to help young people strive to be better and also learn how to overcome obstacles.

Jumping and throwing 10-15 minutes: all-round skills.

This has nothing to do with speed but all of our young athletes try everything. The throwing takes longer due to the recovery of the implements.

Game 5-10 minutes: unwind and express personality.

We play a final game that allows the children to organise and compete in small groups. This could be a relay, a pass-and-catch team effort over 400m, paired hare/ hounds tag, or even dodgeball.

As the children mature and gain confidence and understanding I add a technical point or two in the sessions. I am in no rush to demonstrate my technical knowledge to them. I have learned to be patient and draw upon it when the children have shown that they are receptive and that their bodies are ready for specific work.

I do not want children to drop out from our sessions because the early maturers are winning every race and drill that we do.

26: MENTAL HEALTH IN ADOLESCENT ATHLETES

I am constantly amazed and inspired by how children respond in either our club sessions or the school sessions I teach. Children who come in unfit, clumsy and unskilled are transformed into competent, enthusiastic and creative athletes in only a few weeks.

All they need is some structure, guidance, support and the chance to explore and play with their friends.

However, a recent study of 17,000 adolescent athletes in the USA found that levels of anxiety and depression were higher than before the Covid restrictions and that overall quality of life (QOL) was lower.

This was despite the athletes resuming their sporting and exercise activities.

Coaches and teachers should be aware that even if the young athlete in front of them seems physically competent they might be fragile mentally.
If coaches focus on the Xs and Os without looking after the Janes and the Joes, then they might experience a dropout from their teams and squads.

A fable.

The Greek slave, Aesop told a fable about the North Wind and the Sun seeing a traveller and arguing about who could get him to remove his cloak.

The North Wind blew and blew, but it only made the traveller wrap his cloak tighter and lean into the wind.

I was reminded of this 10 days ago when a bevvy of British politicians did the media rounds denigrating the youth of today when launching their 'National Service' policy.

"They need to toughen up." Grant Shapps (Who has never served in the military or the NHS) said.

"They need to get out of their bubble." James Cleverly (Education secretary for less than 2 months) said, forgetting that the Government told us to be in 'bubbles' during the COVID pandemic.

He also forgot that children were forced to stay home for the first 6 months of the pandemic, unable to see their friends and play in parks outside that had been shut down, while restaurants and pubs reopened. Schools were shut for a second time over the next winter.

Is it any wonder children were anxious about venturing outside and trying new things?

Returning to Aesop's fable, the Sun decided to bask the traveller with warmth. The traveller got hot, removed his cloak and rested in the shade of a tree.

The Sun won the bet.

The Landscape for young athletes has changed.

The widespread cancellation of sporting fixtures and training sessions during the early stages of the Covid pandemic led to unfortunate mental health issues. In a comprehensive survey of adolescent athletes, 37% reported moderate to severe levels of anxiety and 40% reported moderate to severe levels of depression.

The good news was that a year later, in a separate survey, the levels of anxiety had dropped to 17% and depression to 15%. The bad news is that this was much higher than pre-Covid levels. There appears to be a lingering effect on mental health in adolescent athletes despite the return to physical activity.

Coach the person, not the athlete.

This is a coaching mantra that is more important than ever. The idea that a young athlete is a number on a spreadsheet or a pawn in a grand game of coach ego chess is outdated. Taking the person in front of you for granted or treating them purely as an object to achieve titles or medals will likely lead to them underperforming or dropping out of the sport completely.

Many young people prefer video games to real games because they can play with their friends without an adult telling them what to do.

Having empathy with the young athlete does not mean that you are 'soft' (and coaches who think this might question why they are coaching in the first place) but that you care.

"People don't care how much you know until they know how much you care." Teddy Roosevelt.

Simple ways to show that you care are:

Greeting every athlete on arrival or, if a big group all arrive at the same time, greeting them as a group and then speaking to every individual at some point in every session.

'Hello' and 'How are you?' are two of the most effective coaching phrases you can use and are free. Use them.

Ask them something that is non-sport related. 'How is school?' 'Did you have a good weekend?' 'Do you have any plans for the holidays?'

This is a better first interaction with an athlete than, 'You need to catch the ball with your hands,' 'Keep your chest up,' or any other technical points.

Also, be mindful of your body language and where you stand. If you always stand in the same corner, talking to the same group or individual, the others will notice. If you are always looking at your laptop or tablet or talking on your phone, the young athletes will realise you are not paying attention to them.

If the young athletes are made to feel welcome and that you are interested in their well-being as well as their sporting performance, then they are encouraged to stick with the sessions and try to improve.

Warning signs.

As well as adopting (or continuing) best practice ideas as suggested above, coaches should be aware of potential signs of anxiety and depression in young athletes so that they can initiate a discussion with parents and signpost them to professionals who can help.

Anxiety presents itself differently from person to person. There might be some obvious physical signs such as reddening of the skin, shaking and sweating: but these might be hard to distinguish from normal signs of vigorous exercise. Other signs include 'stomach ache,' trouble sleeping and restlessness. If the coach has regular chats with the young athlete (see above) then a change in their demeanour will be easier to spot.

It is unlikely that a young athlete will be able to verbally express, 'I feel anxious.' So asking, 'Are you anxious about something?' is unhelpful.
Signs that might indicate a young athlete is depressed include:

- feeling tired or grumpy
- lacking self-confidence or being more self-critical
- being tearful
- feeling sad, miserable or lonely for a long time
- have trouble sleeping or sleeping more than usual.

- withdrawing from usual activities with friends
- eating less or eating more than usual.
- self-harming

It takes a medical professional to diagnose depression. We can not diagnose it as coaches but we can help the young athlete by discussing with parents if we see some of the warning signs above.

They are not indicators that the young athlete 'lacks commitment' or 'focus.' We should not add misery to their experience by telling them to work harder or to 'snap out of it.' If the young athlete feels anxious or is exhibiting signs of depression and we can help them, then we are acting responsibly.

Mental health is as important as physical health. Coaches should not force injured players to play sports nor should they force or ignore athletes who are suffering from mental health issues.

By treating young athletes as people and supporting them through their troubles, coaches can make a real difference to them. Hopefully, the young athletes can recover and continue their enjoyment of the sport.

27: REFLECTIVE PRACTICE FOR COACHES

Plan, Do, Review is a basic outline of the coaching process. Most coaches love the doing part, some are good at planning, but what about the review? In my experience this is the poor, neglected child of coaching; an afterthought that might be brought up once a year in a formal evaluation setting. It is a bit like a cool down in the training environment, everyone knows it is important, but is too busy or tired to do it properly.

I have used the term reflective practice in the title because it implies introspection and thought about improving oneself, rather than just improving our sessions (although the two are hardly separate in reality). I shall emphasise this for the remainder of the article, rather than looking at what technical/tactical improvements can be made—the 'How' to coach, rather than the 'What' to coach.

"Research has shown experiential learning to be the primary determinant of developing coach expertise." (Knowles et al,1).

In the military the term debrief is used to evaluate missions, a formal environment that can be brutally honest, for others to learn and for overall effectiveness and safety to improve. The airline industry also sets high standards for debriefs after accidents and shares information worldwide to improve safety.

The most important thing is that an evaluation does take place. Without any assessment of what we have done we are in danger of doing the same thing session after session, year after year.

When should we review?

"I don't have time to review," cries the coach, *"I've got to put the cones away, drive to the next venue, call an athlete's mum and organise the minibus for the next tournament."*

There are three times when we can reflect on our practice:

1. In the session- We see an exercise is too hard or too easy for our athlete, so we adjust accordingly. The athlete is injured so we have to devise an alternative to our plan.

2. Post-session- We think about what happened and decide to change something for the next session. Our athletes were unable to receive the bar deep enough when snatching, so we add snatch balance to the next session's warm-up.

3. Post-season- The more formal in-depth review. Did we meet our targets, how many players came and went, and how did we manage the sessions?

In session, reflection happens immediately. The more experienced the coach, the more tools they have in their toolbox, the better they can adjust. The beginner coach often has their plan and sticks rigidly to it. They do not have the ability or confidence to change midway through the session, even if they see something isn't working.

In team sports, the coaches often adjust tactics at half-time; Bill Belichick was the master of this with the New England Patriots. When I assess strength and conditioning coaches in their practice, I often see a desire to stick to the plan. The coach can see something going wrong but is afraid to change. For some reason, the Excel spreadsheet is of more importance than events happening on the ground.

Solutions to the problem can come from different sources if you are open to them.

I saw a potential hazard a few weeks ago when coaching gymnastics where two groups were likely to finish in the same area. I was scratching my head about how to run them concurrently when Archie, a 12–year–old human rubber ball, suggested I change the direction of travel for one of the drills. I thanked him and went with it.

Question: Do you adjust your session plan in the session?

Reflecting on immediate practice.

I used to drive home after a day of coaching, thinking about sessions and what could have gone better, what went well and who was a pain in the butt that day. I would write notes down when I got home and use them when planning the sessions for the next day.

That was before I had children. I soon realised that if I wanted to stay married, I had to relieve my wife of the nappy-changing, tantrum-calming, puke-clearing duties. Two hours later I would collapse in a heap, all thoughts of coaching expunged from my mind. I did tinker with electronic methods of recording and reflecting during these busy times.

I used Evernote because it synchronises between phone, tablet and computer. I could use a voice note walking back to the car knowing it would be on my laptop when I next logged in. This was handy for adjusting the session plan for the next day.

Things are more settled now, so I have gone back to using an A5 coaching journal to write notes down, a purely personal preference. You can write freestyle or use a simple checklist to evaluate your session. Printing out checklists is tedious and environmentally unsound. One possible solution is to print one copy and keep it at the front of your journal as a reminder of which questions to ask yourself.

This could include:

1. Did my session achieve its goals?
2. Did I communicate the session goals with the athletes?
3. Did I allow time for athlete interaction?
4. Did I give athletes a choice?
5. Did I greet each athlete positively?
6. What do I need to adjust for the next session?

This would only take 2 minutes to write down. Your list of questions might be different, depending on what you are trying to achieve within your session.

The end-of-season review.

This should take a bit longer and use information gathered from the previous season. I find doing it immediately after the season too soon. I prefer taking at least a week off to allow a sense of perspective. If you leave it until the week before pre-season however, it may be too late to make changes.

At this point, once a year, introspection about your coaching philosophy is essential.

"Coach education must create opportunities for developing coaches that will enable the coach to move beyond existing practice, to innovate, to experiment, to adapt, to reflect, and to build underpinning knowledge and skills for the requirements of 'higher levels' of coaching." (J Lyle,2).

Asking the right questions is crucial, they may include:

1. Do I enjoy coaching?
2. Am I in the right place?
3. Have I balanced work, health, and family well?
4. Have I developed my technical skills?
5. Have I had satisfying personal relationships?
6. Have I resolved conflict well?

7. How can I improve on the areas above?
8. Who can help me?

I never do this in the usual working environment. There are likely to be distractions or a tendency to conform because the physical surroundings remind us of the norm. I do it somewhere different to allow time and space to think. Take your notes from your end-of-session reviews, plus any other sources of feedback (see below) that you have.

Three sources of information.

Three main sources of feedback can help your reflective practice.

1. **Self-evaluation**: be honest with yourself; take time to do it regularly.
2. **Athlete feedback**: Essential and often surprising.
3. **Peer-to-peer**: useful if you can do it, also known as 'Critical Friendship.'

Do you ask for feedback from your athletes? Is it in the form of "Any questions?" at the end of a session?

Some coaching environments, especially where it is 1:1, do involve a lot of feedback. In others, it is forbidden, or not even contemplated. I have trained in many such environments where the coach was the fount of all knowledge and no one ever dared ask them a question.

Whilst coaches may be used to giving feedback, are they as good at receiving it? We must also consider who is in front of us, giving a formal feedback evaluation form to a 9-year-old is probably inappropriate.

In diagram 1 you can see some responses from our club athletes at the end of one 5-week training block They were aged 9-13 and have been training for some time now. I used an idea from 'Practice Perfect' (3). I gave each athlete a pen and an index card and asked them to write down one thing they liked, and one thing we could improve. The last part was either the session content or how I coached. They then folded the card up and put it into a hat.

They knew the feedback was anonymous, and no one was judging them. I later typed up the responses and used them to change my sessions for the next block.

One thing I liked	One thing I would like to improve
I really liked skipping	I need to work on side step ups
I really liked it when we used the medicine balls and skipping	I need to work on my strength e.g. inverted rows and 4d pro hip locks. We could do more ball work.
I enjoyed doing the 4d pro and the inverted rows.	I would like to be able to get my feet to my hands on hanging leg raises
I liked doing the hanging leg raises each week and I think I improved my strength.	I need to improve my upper body strength for exercises that used upper body strength.
I liked the 4d pro	I would like it if we could have more time.
I have learnt how to stand up straight and the benefits from it. I didn't enjoy the skipping so much as I already know how to do it.	I would like to have more of a range of things to do.
I liked doing the inverted rows and the 4d pro.	I find hanging leg raises hard.
I liked the 4d pro hip lock.	I think we should do more push ups.
I like the silly walks	I need to improve on the hanging leg raises (straight legs).
I enjoy the pull ups because they build up my strength.	I want to carry on with my sprinting technique
I enjoy the leg raises, skipping and 4d pro.	I need to practice my extension.
I liked the step ups and the 4d pro. I improved my timing so now I run faster.	I would like to work on my strength and posture.
I like the step ups because I have big legs to use that to an advantage.	I don't like hanging leg rasies. I need to work on my arms.
I like the 4d pro.	James is my dad.

Diagram 1

As you can see, some of them are conflicting- you can't please everyone- but I gave that feedback to the athletes. They appreciated the response. If you ask people to take the time to give feedback, then have the courtesy to acknowledge them, even if you can't action their request.

I have found this to be easy, informative, and open (I think), and has improved what I do.

Peer-to-peer feedback is a simple concept, but often difficult to achieve in practice. As coaches, we should be able to identify behaviours or areas for improvement and recognise great teaching movements without making them personal.

"Your session rocked man," or *"Those single-legged snatch variations are really cool,"* are only useful as ego massagers rather than effective feedback for a colleague.

Again, using the format from 'Practice Perfect', asking a colleague to tell you one thing that went well, and one thing that could be improved is useful. I do this in every coaching course I run, and it is amazing how difficult this is initially for coaches to give and receive.

But, within a few practices, the feedback is relevant, specific and fast. These microdoses of feedback allow us to make simple changes immediately or at least for us to start trying. This includes things like:

• Body positioning
• Tone of voice
• Answering your own questions
• Talking too much
• Demonstrating and talking simultaneously
• Giving five technical points before allowing the athletes to attempt the task
• Saying 'obviously' before each point

The coach receiving the feedback often does a Homer Simpson "*Doh!*", slaps their forehead and nods in agreement as they recognise how they can improve.

We often need someone to point out what we know but have forgotten or fail to see. When we remove the personal and just point to the action, we get essential information that allows us to reflect and improve our practice.

References.
1. Zoë Knowles, Andy Borrie & Hamish Telfer (2005) Towards the reflective sports coach: issues of context, education and application, Ergonomics, 48:11-14, 1711-1720, DOI: 10.1080/00140130500101288
2. LYLE, J. (2002) Sports Coaching Concepts: A Framework for Coaches' Behaviour (London: Routledge).
3. Lemov, D., Woolway, E. & Yezzi, K. (2012) Practice Perfect: 42 rules for getting better at getting better (San Francisco: Jossey-Bass).

28: SEVEN SPORTS SCIENCE MYTHS

Dr Mike Joyner is a faculty member of the Mayo Clinic specialising in human performance physiology.

I met him early on a Wednesday morning at Rice University in Houston, when he was attempting to roll around on the floor and get up despite his very long levers. What impressed me was his effort and concentration in attempting a new task, no matter how difficult.

We then had a great conversation over breakfast about long-term athlete development, fundamental tumbling skills and education for those from a less-than-ideal background. Fuelled by his enthusiasm and some pancakes and coffee, I was primed to learn his thoughts on sports science.

Here is a summary of the key points from his GAIN seminar about sports science myths:

1. Lactic Acid Makes Me Sore.

Lactic acid is removed in 40/50 minutes post-exercise. Active recovery does help this process, but ALL lactic acid is gone within 24 hours. Soreness after training is due to muscle damage.

2. Sports drinks and glucose are necessary.

There is no effect of glucose ingestion until after 60 minutes of steady-state exercise. Longer duration bouts of exercise may require some. There are many different variables including; the duration and intensity of the bout factors, and the nutritional status before exercise.

Most studies are conducted early in the morning when the athletes are fasting, so extrapolating this to afternoon exercise may be tenuous. The 2% reduction in body weight due to dehydration DOES impact performance, so hydration matters. Rinsing out the mouth with sugar can affect performance positively: it is like "brain candy".

3. It must be genetic.

Size is the obvious example where genetics matter (I would say gender matters more) but there are only a few examples of what Dr Joyner calls 'O. Athletes' (Knockout).

An example of breeding would be Christian McCaffrey (drafted by Carolina

Panthers, currently with the San Francisco 49ers) whose dad was Ed McCaffrey (Giants, 49ers, Broncos) and his maternal grandfather was Dave Sime who was an Olympic silver medallist in the 100m in 1960.

Otherwise, studies have found little evidence for a 'talent gene' except for some with ACTN3 and ACE genotypes for speed. There is no evidence for gene testing in young people to "predict talent".

Dr Joyner said there is a lot of *"lazy thinking"* about genetics. He then showed a slide with the headline:
"There are more mile/ 1500m world record holders from Kansas than Kenya!"

The DNA variables would need to be explained: Energy systems, muscle fibre type, superior coordination, body composition, motivation, psychology and trainability. They would NOT explain social factors.

4. To stretch or not to stretch?

There is a vast amount of evidence on this, and it is all context-specific. I made the point that a lot of the studies are asking the wrong question. *"Does stretching before exercise prevent injury?"* and then tested on military recruits before doing a 20-mile route march with kit in boots. Stretching is the least important factor in that context.

5. Altitude Training.

The 1968 Olympics played a key role in the development of this research as for the first time athletes would be competing at altitude on a big scale. There is a need to compare the short vs long-term effects due to the initial reduction in training quality.

Dr Joyner says the data on Live High- Train Low is *"all over the place."* The long-term effects of living at altitude are an increase in lung capacity. But, you have to keep the training quality up. Those who used altitude training successfully did a lot of short intervals to maintain quality.

Some key points he asked us to consider were:

Beware of individual variation; more is not always better; give it time to work; beware of effects on intensity training and volume; recovery is sometimes affected due to a reduction in sleep quality.

6. My programme is better than your programme!

Dr Joyner showed a video clip of one of the Olympic middle-distance races (I forget which) where the top 3 finishers were very close. All 3 of those runners followed very different training programmes: high mileage or high-intensity intervals and so on. Yet, all 3 were effective.

The idea that one programme is inherently better than another is flawed. In strength training research it isn't so much the number of sets vs reps it's the training to failure that is important. As long as intensity is involved, gains will be made in strength.

Dr Joyner then showed video clips from the 'Miracles of Men' ESPN documentary of the Soviet Ice Hockey team doing some very basic 'old school' training in a gym. The imagination and variety of exercises were novel but the players were working hard too (This clip can also be seen in the Red Army documentary on Netflix).

He also showed the clip of the La Sierra High School training programme of the 1960sand what 15 minutes a day can do to form the foundation that is lacking in today's youth (https://rb.gy/6dfbcr).

7. Today's athletes are better.

More people are competing today, with better financial incentives, so records tend to fall. Doping has also had an impact on some performances too.

However, some of yesteryear's performances were pretty impressive. Don Lash, in the 1930s, set the 2-mile record of 8:58.4 on a weekly mileage total of 25 miles.

He made a comparison between Andre DeGrass and Jesse Owens shows the difference in track and shoes between 1936 and 2011.

Dr Joyner also showed how innovation changed standard practices and protocols. Everyone knows about Dick Fosbury, but at the same time Debbie Brill, a 13-year-old girl, was doing the same technique. Both of them were able to try this because of better landing surfaces on the other side of the bar.

Summary.

In the discussion that followed Dr Joyner summarised with **"Get kids out, have fun, spend time with good coaches."** (That sounds a lot like what we are trying to do at Excelsior ADC).

This was a refreshing and engaging discussion, which I have only briefly touched upon. I spoke to Dr Joyner about academics preaching to each other from Ivory Towers without actually coming into contact with real people in the real world.

He said, *"That's why I practice Medicine one day a week, so I stay in touch."*

29: MICRO-DOSING FOR EFFICIENCY

Except for professional players and undergraduates, most sportspeople are time-poor. Travel, work, study, family and competing all take up time in strangely inconvenient blocks that mess up your meticulous training routine.

If the plan says, '90 minutes', then it is easy to become disheartened when you only have 60 available. Or, for the ultra-committed, you become sleep-deprived as sleep is what 'gives' to 'make it.' This short-term solution comes back to kick you in the backside as you underperform in your sport or life.

Micro-dosing is a simple method of re-framing your perception of time, allowing you to work within frequent, smaller periods. It solves some of the problems and may enhance certain aspects of your training. I shall outline some of the pros and cons in this article and how I have used them.

Re-framing your goals.

Roger Bannister was a med-student when he broke the 4-minute mile. He only had an hour to train daily, and his sporting goal matched his available time.

Compare that with recreational runners whose goal is to run a half-marathon: big mileage is required, and if you are running slowly, this takes up more time. Distance is king and everyone is trying to do more. But running 80 miles a week leaves you too mentally and physically tired to do much else.

If you are genuinely time-poor, the first thing to do is set a goal that matches the available time. This reduces anxiety and you are more likely to achieve your new goal.

For example, the recreational runner who jogs 8-minute miles might try this:
· Previous goal: run a half-marathon.
· New goal: run a mile in less than 6 minutes.

For this runner, the overall volume would decrease and the type of training would change: more sprints and intervals rather than long runs. This could be accomplished in less training time.

Setting up your training plan.

What are your essentials?

Write down what you 'need to do,' compared to what is 'nice to do'. Imagine you only had 15 minutes a day, what would you do? I use 15-minutes because it focuses your mind on what matters most (N.B. If you write down, 'foam-roller', try again).

For example, it might be for a weightlifter:
· Snatch
· Cleans
· Jerks
· Squats

For the 8-min mile runner who is trying to get to 6-min miles it might be:
· 1.5-mile run
· 3 x800m @3:45 pace with 1-minute rest.
· 6 x 200m @ 45-second pace with 1:45 rest

Once you have this, 'need-to-do' you can expand from there. You might have a couple of 15-minute chunks a day rather than a 30-minute block, so the weightlifter might snatch in the morning and squat in the afternoon.

This is simply a matter of changing your mindset from, '*I need an hour to train,*' to '*What can I get done?*' This is more easily written than implemented.

Office working and student runners beware of high-speed running in a short time. I have seen many people get calf injuries after spending a morning sitting at a desk with their legs tucked behind them and then trying to run fast. If you can, move around your office or sit in a different position before running. You might try starting with walking to jogging to run rather than straight into running.

It is unlikely that 15 minutes a day will lead you to improved performance, and so, at some point, you will need more time. This might be at the weekends or on alternate days. The important point is not to squander that time with fluff. Use it to do your maximum lifts, long runs, or speed sessions where you need long rest intervals.

However, if you are in a busy period such as exams, work deadlines, or having a newborn baby, doing 15 minutes a day might not improve performance but it can prevent a precipitous decline.

Can you micro-dose at home?

The second element of micro-dosing is the 'homework' aspect of training for the recreational athlete. Many sportspeople train twice a week with the club and play a match at the weekend. The coach is limited in time in practice and so devotes 95% of this time to technical and tactical work. Fitness and individual skills are left out.

I have used many variations of micro-dosing to help athletes work on what is left out in training, but they all come back to two questions:

1. Does the athlete want to train?
2. How can I make it accessible and interesting?
I am still working on the latter.

As my knowledge of exercises has improved alongside the improvement in technology, filming short exercise clips and sharing them, has become a lot easier. I still recommend 5-10 minutes a day and give a list of exercises to complete each week.

I don't like the 'Monday; lunges, Tuesday: Heel slides,...' prescriptive approach because every athlete has a different schedule and life throws curve balls that often scupper Monday's plan.

If I give 6 'micro-sessions' to complete, then the athlete can do one a day or two for three days.

My best guess is to give some structure to athletes that allow room for adapting to their schedules. They must be coached through the exercises and be familiar with them. Barriers and obstacles to 'getting it done' should be discussed. I always get the athletes to give me a when and where and describe how they are going to do it.

Most people fail on the 'how to fit it in', not the 'what should I do?'

Here are two micro-dose sessions and you can see how I am coaching the athletes before giving it as homework.

- Squat mobility (https://rb.gy/eoamd7).

- 'Strength and flex' (https://rb.gy/jv7zjy).

Remember, the point is not to impress our coaching peers with our fancy programmes but to help our athletes improve.

A handwritten note with a stick man drawing, that the athlete does diligently, is better than the 20-page document that gathers virtual dust.

Summary.

Life is tough and we need to realise that we can't do everything all of the time. But, if we reframe our goals, narrow down what is essential and build some adaptability into our training, we can make our sporting life a little easier.

30: WHY PE SHOULD BE MORE 'WE' THAN 'ME'

"Children need to express themselves as individuals."

So goes modern thought as we create a generation of self-centred, narcissistic kids who are unable to cope with failure when it happens. Adults have allowed mega-corporations to inflict their addictive programmes onto children via smartphones.

With mental health issues, including loneliness and isolation, prevalent in society, is now a time for a more cooperative approach to physical activity?

Politicians create culture wars rather than develop long-term strategies to improve our country and benefit the citizens. Or worse, they remove effective policies such as 'Sure Start' because it wasn't their idea!

'Strivers versus Skivers' was one horrible phrase used by politicians to create disharmony amongst our population and there are many others.

But what if children lack support, guidance and opportunity to learn and improve? The erstwhile 'strivers' soon become disillusioned and realise that their effort leads to frustration so they quit.

Politicians who have little understanding of Physical Education could be part of the problem. They create PE curricula based on either adult-led competitive sports or a 'let's just get them moving' mantra.

P.E. classes in the teenage years have become less about doing, and more about 'theory of doing.' Children can recite the five elements of fitness but can't touch their toes, let alone do a handstand. Then we send them out to play 15-a-side rugby.

We now have a generation of p.e. teachers who came through this system and are now teaching children with their limited knowledge. A female p.e. teacher told my 14-year-old son that he was squatting wrong (i.e. full-depth) and should know better because his dad was a coach!

He was doing a full range of motion that few teenagers can manage thanks to their school-acquired deformities and too much time on screens.

As to girls, lots of schools have thrown their hands up in the air and think that sticking them on Wii. or a Cross trainer watching TV. is the way forward. One of our club athletes was asked, 'Why are you doing weightlifting?' by the deputy head of her school.

I don't understand why p.e. teachers feel the need to denigrate those pupils who are active and might know more than they do!

Physical education can be divided into three basic content areas.

(According to Dr Ed Thomas of the Iowa Health and Physical Readiness Alliance in Chapter 6 of his book Rama).

1. Restorative–Techniques, obvious or subtle, that bring the body toward its optimal state of harmony and compensate for the stress of daily life.

2. Martial–Techniques, obvious or subtle, that teach appropriate offensive and defensive responses to external aggression.

3. Pedagogical–Sports, games, theoretical bodies of knowledge, and dance.

Instead of using all three content areas, dance, theory and games form the Modern Pedagogical part of Physical Culture: where are the Martial and Restorative components?

Without the other areas, we are creating content like a one-legged stool.

The function of physical education can also be divided into three areas.

1. Personal-The focus of this aspect is on individual health, comfort, and physical gratification. Here the self is felt to exist at the borders of the skin and the limits of personal desire. It can easily be reduced to self-indulgence but can also serve to stimulate healthy life habits.

2. Interpersonal–At this level, one's attention turns to the needs of others. At lower levels, it may be confined to family, neighbourhood, gender, race, and so forth. Higher development brings awareness that all able citizens must be physically and mentally prepared to defend the highest ideals of their nation and to contribute productively to its future.
Further growth will lead to the realization that national borders are superficial boundaries within an interdependent family of living organisms who share the earth.

3. Transpersonal–Cultures vary greatly in the development and understanding of obvious and subtle physical techniques that contribute to the spiritual quest. Transcendence brings the uninterrupted, moment-to-moment realisation that all things are divinely One.

Any or all of the following can increase power:

Increasing the force applied. $P = (Fd)/t$

Increasing the distance travelled. $P = (fD)/t$

Reducing the time it takes. $P = (fd)/T$

Or, a combination of all three.

For example, when driving down with the plant leg in sprinting, we want to increase the force and reduce the time the foot spends on the ground, this creates more power and the sprinter runs faster.

Or, in throwing events, we can increase the distance the implement travels (shot, discus) by adding more turns or half turns, and reducing the time taken to cover this distance by turning faster, this increases the power and acceleration at release.

Jim Radcliffe uses the terms, Resistive, Spatial and Temporal Overload to categorise different exercises.

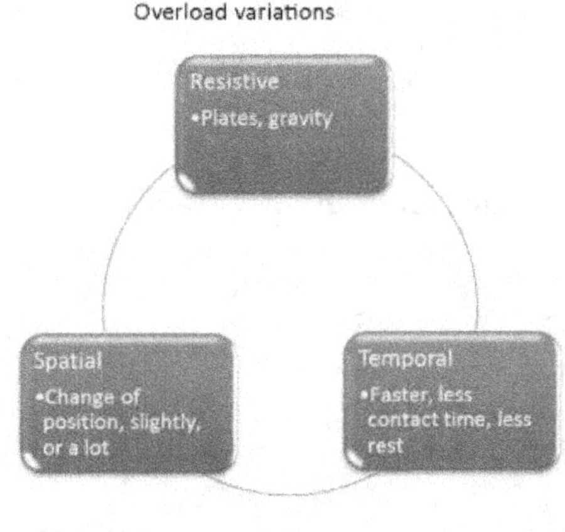

Excelsior, with thanks to Jim Radcliffe.

www.excelsiorgroup.co.uk

Remember that **Power = Force x distance/ time.** $P=(fd)/t$

The 3 overload variations are:

Resistive: using gravity or external resistance (f)

Spatial: train outside of the platform, small variations leading to big ones (d).

Temporal: do the same work but faster, with less rest, or less contact time (t)

When planning training programmes, it is best to focus on one aspect at a time, whilst maintaining the others.

For example:
A fencer must be able to cover big distances, fast, with little or no external resistance, except gravity and air. Working on spatial and temporal overload makes sense, rather than resistive overload (badminton, squash, tennis and volleyball have similar requirements).

The lateral circuit in this video (https://rb.gy/9mu0qa) is for a field hockey player and is designed to help spatial and temporal aspects. The resistive force is minimal (body weight).

Conversely, a tight head prop has to overcome massive external resistance in both the scrum and in the contact areas. It makes sense to concentrate on resistive overload, rather than spatial overload (although the latter is always amusing). American football linemen have similar requirements but also need to be able to pull/trap get downfield.

Unfortunately, it is common to see a 'one-size-fits-all' approach when trying to develop power.

The relationship between force, distance and time.

Whilst there needs to be a different emphasis at any one time, all three components are interrelated. It is difficult to cover more distance (spatial) without the ability to produce force. That can be aided by resistive training. Similarly, having great strength, without the ability to move fast, or cover distance is often useless in the sporting environment.

The problem occurs in training environments where one is the focus to the exclusion of all else. One example was that British fencers were told they had to be able to squat and deadlift twice their body weight! This shows a complete lack of imagination and understanding of what the sport requires.

Yes, most fencers could be stronger and need to be, but that has to apply to what their sporting requirements are rather than what matches the sports scientists' manual.

Part of the problem was that many sports scientists saw an opportunity to data mine the complicit athletes to gain PhDs! Once they became a 'Doctor', the sports scientists left the NGB and the athletes to pick up the broken pieces (Ethics: discuss).

Practical ideas to develop power without weights.

Before increasing the speed or distance or volume of exercises, ensure decent form and good control. Power is useless without control. Being injured won't help you get more powerful either.

When thinking about distance, think about direction too. It is easy to be restricted by the lifting platform or power rack. Instead, think up, down, left and right, forward and back and combinations of all of these.

Here are some examples:

In this simple warm-up (https://rb.gy/yh5p1v) the weightlifters are going over and under the hurdles. Their hips have to fully extend and then fully flex.

This series of lunge exercises (https://rb.gy/fc1jfp) challenges the distance in different directions and by adding the dumbbells, the distance between fingernails and toenails. Racquet sports such as tennis and badminton require the players to extend legs and arms together. This helps prepare them for that.

Speed exercises.

In this skipping drill (https://rb.gy/vleii1), the distance the foot travels increases but the cadence remains the same. The leg has to move faster to accomplish the task. Drills like this help train the components of running which can then be put together immediately afterwards into sprinting.

This toe jump drill (https://rb.gy/20jzu2)is designed to reduce the time spent on the ground when running. The foot has to be pulled up and actively whipped down. Feel that the big toes are pointing upwards as you land: that helps tense the tendons in the foot arch and they react with more spring.

Applying the power equation to your session design.

Once the athletes understand what we are trying to achieve, their focus and effort are applied in the right direction. They know whether we are trying to go heavier (force), faster (speed) or further (distance).

I have shown four examples of exercises and explained why they are used.

Once you understand why, you can apply the principle to many other exercises. For example:

Squats. Put on a disco song (120 bpm) and try to do one bodyweight squat per second (start with 10). One beat is up, the next beat is down. That is twice as fast as you would normally move.

Skipping: skip ten times and try to cover as much distance as possible. Next, see how many foot contacts you can get within 10 metres (moving faster).

Conclusion.

When setting out your plan, look at the athlete's strengths and weaknesses, compare that to the sporting requirements, and adjust accordingly.
The 3 types of overload may help you start to systemise what you do and why.

"The best way to get better?.... is to get smarter!" Jim Radcliffe.

32: ARE YOU TEACHING OR TESTING?

Strength and Conditioning coaches often deal with a captive market who are forced to 'engage'. This can result in less-than-ideal practices: the coaches can get away with things because the athletes must comply if they want to get selected for a team or squad.

For example, 13-year-old girls who want to play golf will only be doing 8 RM back squats because they are forced, rather than because they choose.

Physical education teachers must create an environment and lesson structure that generates an active interest in a non-volunteer cohort. Their lessons have to show progression, precision and variety. They have had contact with the children for many years in a row. A child will be in school for about 13 years, longer than they will be with a single coach, or possibly a sport.

Whilst the S&C coach can judge their status by the success of the top athlete or team with whom they work, the PE teacher is judged by the results of all the children in their class. If the S&C coach applied some of the soft skills and sound practices developed within physical education, they might find that all their athletes improved, rather than just the highly motivated few.

The problem with sports science.

I have undertaken two S&C accreditation processes: one in the UK, and one from the USA. Both times I had to spend a lot of time revising sports science and training theory. The exams reflected this.

The first question I had to answer in one was, **"*What is the purpose of a bone notch?*"**

It went downhill from there.

Whilst I passed both exams on my first attempt, I never felt that I was a better 'coach'. Instead, I knew a lot of information (at least I thought I did). I only had to conduct one small coaching session with another person during the whole accreditation process: the rest was just theory.

My impression of sports science is that it focuses a lot on measuring and monitoring. This transfers to the S&C culture of testing and benchmarks. Training sessions are reverse-engineered from the desired number. These numbers become very important and are shared with other people. The S&C coach or sports scientist may have their performance benchmarked by the measurements of the athletes trained.

The most important aspect of coaching is the interaction between human beings. If we start to see athletes as numbers, rather than people, we can easily fall into the trap of just measuring and monitoring rather than teaching. Compounding this trait is the rise of the super-facility. Power platforms, watt bikes and bar-velocity tags mean that if it moves, it's measured.

Forget about the quality of movement, we need a number.

Compare that to the daily life of a PE teacher who has 30 children in a class with minimal equipment and limited time in which to teach. If that teacher has only got a sports science degree and then has done a one-year PGCE to become 'teacher-trained,' they may well get a shock to find out that the pupils respond in a random, chaotic fashion, rather than sit diligently waiting to be measured.

The Broad Jump.

The broad jump is frequently used to assess an athlete's ability to demonstrate power. I have been told many times by NGBs to get a number for each of the athletes that I coach. Often I have been told to do this on Day 1 of meeting the person (they are a person, remember).

"Hi, I am James, I need to get a number from you. I don't care about your dreams, aspirations, background, experience, problems and life. Stand here and jump."

The athlete jumped, I measured, they repeated it twice more, and I recorded and sent the data to the NGB. We all congratulated ourselves on 'a job well done.'

Two weeks later the athlete has not got any better and I am then told to have a conversation about their 'lack of engagement.'

That is not how I approach the broad jump now. Greg Thompson pointed me the way to Educational Gymnastics. Along that route, I found a useful piece about guided discovery and jumping.

The broad jump is a 2-foot to 2-foot action. There are four other possible foot combinations (each of which has multiple variants). You can see me coaching this here (https://rb.gy/fokhhp).

This has some advantages over just testing:
 • I can observe how the athletes move and whether they can jump and land safely or competently.

- They get to lead their own discovery, automatically developing "engagement".
  - They can do a lot of repetitions without doing too many of any one thing.
  - They learn by doing.

The assumption that every athlete is a competent mover and can perform a maximal effort jump (and landing) test is an assumption too far for me, no matter what their sporting level.

By using some skills gained from physical education, I can help the athlete learn to move and build trust and rapport with them. This trust has to be earned and I need to work hard to create a safe and positive environment for them rather than be another authority figure with a tape measure and clipboard.

This doesn't mean I am trying to be 'down with the kids,' rather I am making an effort to understand what life is like in their shoes.

After a few sessions of developing their jumping, including some exercises where we 'see how far you can jump,' I can then get a tape measure out and record their maximal effort. I am still uncertain as to what this tells me, other than the obvious, but we can then help the athlete develop their jumping ability and remeasure later.

Summary.

Kelvin Giles uses the phrase 'Random Number Gatherers' to describe people with clipboards (or tablets) who measure athletes. It is no surprise that many athletes respond indifferently or reluctantly to being treated as a number.

Using sound teaching principles from physical education, coaches can develop their athletes and improve their performance measures simultaneously.

33: DON'T BE CRUEL TO KITTENS (OR CHILDREN)

An experiment involving two kittens was conducted in a lab in the early 1960s (1). The kittens were put on a small carousel that rotated with a view of the lab. Kitten A could move its feet and the carousel spun as it walked. Kitten B was suspended in a box that rotated to give the same view of the lab that Kitten A had. Kitten B's little paws never touched the box. He just hung and rotated.

When the kittens were released, Kitten A could navigate its surroundings and move around obstacles. Kitten B kept bumping into things and had no sense of body awareness. Poor kitty…

If you have any sense of empathy you will feel for poor Kitten B. You might even feel outraged and think, 'How dare they?' You might jump on Facebook to 'dislike' the research scientists.

Rightly so? Kittens need to be able to explore, search and learn about the environment so that they can cope in the real world.

And yet….

Do you drive your child to school?

Do you drive your child from one organised activity to another?

Are you a Head Teacher who reduces break times and disallows playground games because of 'health and safety'?

If you have said, 'yes' to any of the above, then you are replicating the kitten experiment with your child.

They are likely to grow up like Kitten B: not understanding where their body is in space and how to manipulate it around and over obstacles.

I see this all the time when young children are brought to our gymnastics club. Some have great movement awareness (not specific gym skills) and can coordinate their arms and legs. Others look like they have never been outdoors or walked further than TV to the fridge and back.

You wouldn't do it to a kitten, so why are you driving your child to a school when they could walk, cycle or take the bus which at least requires them to walk to the bus stop?

Parents say things like, 'Oh, she's naturally uncoordinated'.

I believe that coordination, rhythm, timing, physical strength and balance can be taught and developed in EVERY child. If they are given the right opportunity, shown some ideas and allowed to explore in their own time: just like Kitten A.

But what about P.E.?

Are you a P.E. teacher who forces children to sit in queues and listen to your lectures?

A recent study in the UK for year 7 and year 8 pupils showed that they were only 'moderately' or 'vigorously' active for 30% of the time in their PE lessons. That means for 70% of the limited time that they are in P.E. they are not 'doing'.

P.E. teachers: take a hard look at yourselves and change what you are doing. Rounders and cricket are standing around activities. Easy to put on the curriculum and easy to supervise but they are doing little to nothing to help children develop physical skills.

The problem is that P.E. teachers are unaccountable for the physical skills and fitness of the children at school. There are no mandatory tests or guidelines like there are for maths and English. The exception is swimming.

Instead, P.E. departments are measured on their GCSE (academic) results that only a few pupils undertake. Or, they hide behind a competitive sports fixture list that keeps the teachers busy but only a minority of pupils undertake.

Solutions.

It's not about money, resources and facilities. It's about imagination, purpose and consistency.

Encourage children to walk (skip, hop, gallop) to school: parents can then get some exercise too.

Have local parks with safe bicycle and walking access (ditto).

Develop physical education lessons that physically educate the children rather than trying to emulate adult-organised sports.

Stop following lesson plans that say, *'Today is cricket, explain the rules and organise a game,*' that results in two children doing lots of things and the rest standing around getting bored.

Instead; use one of Andy Stone's warm-ups for 5-7 minutes before each lesson to help develop their physical literacy. Here is an example (https://rb.gy/y3qws0).

Then do some general skill and games work that involves pairs and threes rather than 15-a-side and finally have a cricket tournament at the end of the lesson block.

Or, do nothing and watch our children end up like poor little Kitten B.

References.

1 Held, R., & Hein, A. (1963). Movement-produced stimulation in the development of visually guided behavior. Journal of Comparative and Physiological Psychology, 56(5), 872–876 https://doi.org/10.1037/h0040546

2. Beale N, Eldridge E, Delextrat A, et al. Exploring activity levels in physical education lessons in the UK: a cross-sectional examination of activity types and fitness levels. BMJ Open Sport & Exercise Medicine 2021;7:e000924. doi:10.1136/ bmjsem-2020-00092

34: INDIVIDUALISATION IN GROUP ENVIRONMENTS

To paraphrase Kelvin Giles, '*If your coach: athlete ratio is 1:25 then you are managing a crowd, not coaching.*'

Some coaches can only dream of that ratio because they regularly manage groups of 40 or 50 people in a session. In large groups, individualisation may seem impossible and we have to hope that everyone gets some improvement.

Even when I coach an athlete in 1:1 sessions I question how much individualisation of the training programme I can do without a supporting staff of data analysts and sports scientists. There are things we can do as coaches to help individualise the training programme and some things that might be exaggerated. I have more questions than answers but I hope to provoke your thinking.

What is individualisation?

I suggest that "**Individualisation is tailoring your coaching to meet the individual's needs.**"

We first need to identify what the needs are. This is easy to write on paper but harder to do in practice. The questions I ask myself are related to:
   • Age/stage of the athlete.
   • Their sport.
   • Their position.
   • The tactical requirements of their current team.
   • Injury history.
and comparing these to where they want to be in a certain time frame: a week, a month, a year or four years.

So far, so simple. But gathering the information and turning it into a meaningful programme is difficult. Multiplying that out by 10 or 20 players we start to lose the thread and resort to more general principles of training that we perceive as 'truths'.

Scientificy Programming.

The doubts in my mind begin with the methods of gathering data and then translating that into a programme. In a team sport such as football, players wearing GPS devices is very helpful for providing specific information about total work, top speeds, accelerations and changes of direction. GPS can also be worn in training to replicate/ measure the same factors. Twenty years ago, a similar methodology was used with heart rate monitors.

The information gathering has improved, but what do we do with it? The one thing we don't know is how a player will respond to the training stimulus that we use. We guess.

Quoting research studies that show average improvements of a cohort of subjects that have little resemblance to the athlete in front of you does not make sense to me. The gap between data and individualisation widens when we start to use supplementary exercises such as back squats or watt bikes to train footballers. We test and measure the work done in those modes and show 'improvements' but then how has that translated to the sport? Have we individualised the training but not thought about specificity?

Factors that might change an individual's response to any training programme (and this is what we are after the response, not the programme) include:
- Diet
- Hydration status
- Sleep
- Outside stressors
- Age
- Menstrual cycle
- Additional extras (they could be training for the beach at home).
- Demands of the match/ tactical training sessions.

These external factors reign in any chance of me 'guaranteeing' success with an athlete. There are so many variables that it makes my head spin. Whole industries have arisen and National Governing Bodies have spent millions of pounds creating and supporting the measurer and the gadget-maker of widgets that provide the answers.

I don't have that time or budget and at some point, I have to get out and coach.

What can we do to coach the individual?

Looking beyond the physiology for a moment we can get to know the athlete as an individual. Just as every athlete will respond differently to 5 sets of 5 reps of back squats at 80% 1RM, every athlete responds differently to your coaching style. Some need encouraging and constant feedback. Some respond to a direct coaching cue as if you had insulted their maternal bloodline. Some athletes like being asked questions, and some shrivel and blush and feel 'picked on'. Some might like the comfort of a group hug pre-match, while others hate being touched.

It is distinguishing and identifying what works with whom that makes coaching so challenging and interesting for me. We coach humans, not Excel spreadsheets.

No matter how big your squad, every athlete should be greeted and given an individual acknowledgement at some point. This starts with knowing their names. I remember that eight months after being selected for the England Karate Squad (there were ten of us), the head coach asked me halfway through a training session, *"What's your name again?"* There was me trying my hardest and then realising my efforts were undeserving of recognition!

There are assessment tools for gathering information about athletes' psychological profiles and then adapting your coaching to them. I have used some, but I have always found that the pen and paper add another barrier between coach and athlete. Conversations still work best for me. I don't know how to interpret and then act upon 30 sets of profiles. If we delegate that to the sports psychology department, then what are we doing as coaches?

Returning to coaching, when I coach gymnastics, I have 16 people in a group and that feels like a lot. I have one assistant coach. The 1:8 ratio still feels like a lot. We can't have 16 people doing individual programmes so we have to compromise, which I think is where most coaches are.

The session would look like this:

Group: Free practice for 5 minutes (individual choice)
.

Group: Warm up for 5 minutes general, then a sequence of basic skills, for 5-minutes. Individuals can choose within the second section, i.e. 'Forward rolls, any leg variation,' or, 'Cartwheel followed by any other move.'

Stations: Class divided into 4 groups of 4 in roughly similar ability or friendship groups (the latter is as important as the former for these gymnasts: it's not 'high performance', it's social). Here the individualisation is hit and miss. We give choices at some stations such as in vaulting or floor work, but in others it is just a circuit of preparation exercises for harder skills such as somersaults or handsprings that everyone will do.

Pairs: choreographed routine or ideas for them to extrapolate. Here I will show them some skills and a new linking exercise. They then create their own routine or build on from the previous session. I can then offer advice and support according to their needs. Some can work well, while others need help with creativity.

These sessions are far from perfect and there will be times when every gymnast is doing something they don't like or that is well within their skill set. The choice I have to make when planning and implementing is to allow at least some portion of the class for their choice, and another part to cover skills gaps that I identify when reviewing the sessions or that they ask for.

Summary.
It might be possible to tailor your coaching to the individual where the support staff outnumber the athletes. It is hard to do when the coach is outnumbered. As long as the coach is honest and upfront about what is possible and tries to individualise where possible, athletes can be realistic in their expectations and improvements can be made.

35: IMPROVE YOUR COACHING THROUGH STORYTELLING

Ever wondered why you aren't getting through to your athletes or peers? You have listed the references, provided the data, and shown a few charts, just like your undergraduate lecturers told you to. They would be proud.

Professor Bill McGuire, of UCL, said this:

"Scientific papers, however well-written, rarely carry the emotional weight of a good story. Stories have been the prime means of imparting knowledge and warnings throughout human history. Even in today's data-rich world, they hold a visceral clout that no amount of graphs, charts or figures can replace.2 (New Scientist #3372).

And there aren't many well-written scientific papers!

Do you doubt this? Think of The Bible: it's full of stories and parables that stand the test of time (I'm not a Christian but I can remember many of the stories).

Will anything you say and do stick in the memories of the people you are trying to influence as much as the tale of The Good Samaritan?

Chief Storyteller.

Sweden doesn't think so. Its Viable Cities project has hired Per Grankvist to help influence the population to become Carbon-Neutral by 2030.
His job title? Chief Storyteller.

"When it comes to climate change, storytelling is much more important than the transmission of facts. Just bombarding people with facts doesn't work, and neither does shaming people." (The Big Issue #1498).

Grankvist writes stories that show how people might be living in 2030.

Boring people, doing boring things, just like me and you. It's a human touch that we can relate to.

Every coaching course that I have ever attended has stressed the importance of communication. But they seem to talk about different forms of transmitting data, rather than the nuts and bolts of whether the athletes receive, understand and then desire to change.

Storytelling with your athletes.

I don't gather up the young gymnasts that I coach, sit them around the
fireplace and read them a story of Hercules or The Great Gama.
I do use examples of how people have overcome obstacles and how they
managed to change and learn a new skill.

In our club's Instagram posts, I try to share who the people are in the videos
and a little of their background. We emphasise that these aren't superhumans,
they are ordinary Joes and Janes trying to do extraordinary things.

In our club newsletters, I share a longer piece at the beginning of each month,
an idea I took from Arnold Schwarzenegger's excellent newsletter. The theme
is always the same: our club was set up to help young people develop over the
long term. We are there to support and encourage them on their journey
rather than win this Saturday.

Parents are living day to day, week to week, crawling towards the school
holidays when they have to juggle childcare. They don't need facts about
thousands of hours of training and periodised training plans (who does?).
But, seeing a child, or an adult just like them, and hearing their stories, might
help influence them.

I am like King Canute, fighting against the tide of step-counting, early
specialisation, bodybuilding, fad diets and mindless jogging that is endemic in
our society. And that's just the p.e. teachers!

So, telling stories helps explain what we do and why.
What stories can help explain what you do? Think Flash Fiction rather than
Tolstoy.

Be succinct, omit unnecessary words, and be genuine. The stories are there to
help your athletes, not to impress your peers on social media.

Here's an example of me using storytelling to introduce a healthy eating plan
for athletes (https://rb.gy/epsvk2).

36: FROM TEXT BOOK TO NOTE BOOK

In my first MSc in Sports Coaching lecture at Brunel University, we were told to look up super-compensation theory for our homework. The following week the lecturer asked if anyone could explain it, I put my hand up and was asked to stand at the front of the class to draw it on the whiteboard.

"Teacher's pet," said one of my fellow students as I sat down.

The book that I read that week was Tudor Bompa's 'Periodization: Theory and Methodology of Training.'

It included a nice graphic of the super-compensation cycle I had replicated on the class whiteboard. As earnest, mature students we discussed the theories in the book at break time in the refectory and I ordered a copy for my own use as I thought I had hit pay-dirt with the organisation and structure laid out. A few years later I got my copy signed by Mr Bompa after his presentation at a UKSCA conference.

That was then. Now, the once revered tome sits on a shelf gathering dust. The hope and promise of a life made easy following structured plans have been replaced by exasperation and frustration as hundreds of beautifully crafted Excel spreadsheets lie unopened, redundant after coming into contact with the harsh realities of life.

Whilst I have not thrown away the idea of planning, I have discarded the idea that you can plan in detail more than two weeks in advance. I shall now list some examples of how and why I have changed my practice.

Swallowing the periodisation hype.

Back in 2004, I wrote an article for Peak Performance magazine called 'Advanced Periodization Strategies.' I read several research articles on strength gains made using different types of Periodization plans. This was when I was working within professional rugby and was keen to use the most effective types of programmes for the players.

I outlined the results gained from Linear Periodization and Non-Linear Periodization, Reverse Linear Periodization, and Daily Undulating Periodization. The studies all used male college students over 12-15 weeks (nicely fitting into a college semester).

The Daily Undulating Periodization (DUP) looked like this:

Day	Mon	Wed	Mon	Wed
Squat	3sets 10 reps 70% 1RM	5sets 5reps 80% 1RM	6 sets 2 reps 90% 1RM	3sets 10 reps 70% 1RM
Bench Press	3sets 10 reps 70% 1RM	5sets 5reps 80% 1RM	6 sets 2 reps 90% 1RM	3sets 10 reps 70% 1RM
Lunge	3sets 10 reps 70% 1RM	5sets 5reps 80% 1RM	6 sets 2 reps 90% 1RM	3sets 10 reps 70% 1RM
Clean & Jerk	3 sets 5 reps 70%1RM	5sets 3reps 80%1RM	6 sets 1rep 95%1RM	3 sets 5 reps 70%1RM

The 4 exercises remained the same and the sets/reps were manipulated to develop hypertrophy, strength and power and then repeat.

I found the premise of working on three different strength aspects in the same week a manageable process with Academy rugby players 16-18 years old who were playing 1 match a week. I did not use the clean and jerk to help develop hypertrophy, nor the lunge to develop power. I used several different exercises to supplement what we were doing on the day such as squat jumps on the 'power' day and bent over rows on the 'hypertrophy' day.

Because the rugby matches were on the same day each week and I was in a good situation with the rugby coaches who were good planners (and communicators), planning was simple.

What I couldn't understand was how anyone could work on those percentages for more than one week.

How can you test 1RM on the lunge safely? The players either got stronger or more efficient and did not stay lifting the same weights. I adapted the loads according to how they felt on the day. We did our version of Borg's Rating of Perceived Exertion: 'The 9th and 10th rep should feel heavy,' rather than try and calculate the percentages.

I was already modifying what I had read in research into a more coherent training plan that reflected my observations of the players in front of me.

You may think that I am stating the blindingly obvious and yet I attended two UKSCA events during this period where two 'experts' presented their observations and reflections on using a periodized plan with 'elite' athletes.

One worked with an Olympic squad in the USA, the other was an academic who was critiquing coaches' programmes as part of a CPD event. In both events, I saw a complex Excel spreadsheet presented that showed percentages and phrases such as 'speed-strength' used over an annual cycle.

I asked the same question to the experts, *"Is that the plan or the actual lifts done?"*

Both experts answered, *"It is the plan and the actual lifts."*

These experts had somehow managed to find a squad of athletes who could perform every lift for every rep at the exact percentages they had been prescribed up to a year in advance!

If this was the 'expected' and the 'normal' course of events that was being presented by 'experts' then I was failing as a coach. I was always having to chop and change according to how players felt. Either my plan wasn't good enough or maybe, just maybe, what was being presented in conferences and perhaps in the research, was inaccurate.

In my PP article, I wrote a paragraph that was becoming more relevant as I became more experienced:

"Why it may not work."
Standard periodization does not take into account that fixation on sets/ reps/ load does not always mean that a quantifiable training result occurs- other factors are important such as the athlete's perception of the intensity, fatigue, non-training stressors, circadian rhythms as well as the technical / tactical sport sessions all have an effect on the outcome.

Working in an unstable environment.

A couple of years later I was working in a school environment rather than an academy. Here the weeks were longer (6 days of school), the school days were longer and the demands on the pupils were greater. Because the matches were on different days and 'House Matches' of sports such as squash or soccer took place on 'rest days' it was nigh on impossible to programme a DUP.

Instead, I opted for a weekly undulating programme that allowed me to plan for the weeks (Table 2). This meant that if a pupil was only available for 2 sessions in the first week and 3 in the second week, I could keep track of the theme rather than try to juggle 30 different plans.

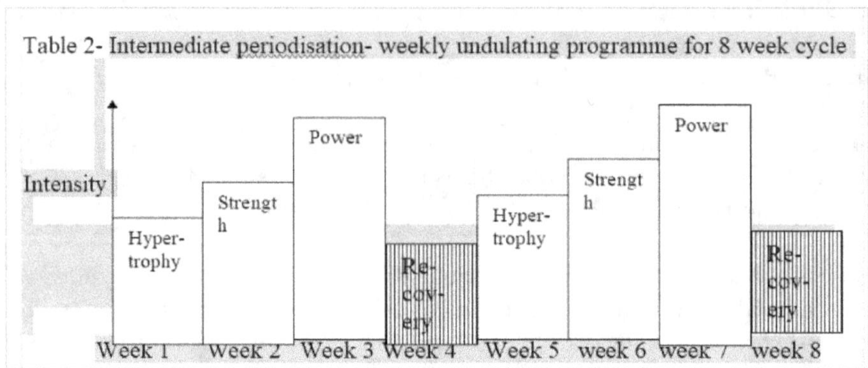

I took a long time planning the sessions for the term by sport, by schedule and by incorporating the gym availability. Each term started on a Monday and the longest that a plan stayed in place before I had to start swapping sessions and exercise was the Tuesday lunchtime.

If we got that far we were doing well.

The school teachers and coaches were not good communicators and many did not understand the point of planning. I was standing waiting with my assistant coach for the rugby team one lunchtime at the beginning of term. This was to be their introduction to the new exercises and an appraisal of how they were moving. They didn't show.

I saw the rugby coach later that afternoon and asked what happened.
"Oh, it was sunny so I thought I would take them on the pitch," he said.

Later that year, the same thing happened. I managed to track the players down: they were taking turns on the Concept II rowers in another gym. The assistant rugby coach was supervising them,
"Why aren't they with me?" I said.
"We have a sevens match on Wednesday so I am getting them fit before that," he said.

I walked outside and bashed my head repeatedly on a convenient brick wall.

On Friday the same teacher came to me and asked if I could do some stretches with the boys instead of weights because *"They've pulled a lot of hamstrings."*

I use those examples to show that no matter how much you plan you can not predict human behaviour.

I learnt to create a framework of what I wanted to achieve but have flexible plans within that. Gary Winckler, at a GAIN conference, said that he never planned more than 2 weeks in detail. It simply wasn't worth it.

How then do the periodization experts manage it?

Groundhog day.

About 10 years ago a new breed of middle management appeared within National Governing Bodies in the UK: the 'lead strength and conditioning coach.' This person was responsible for collating and organising all the individual S&C coaches who worked with athletes or teams within that sport.

Previously I would have communicated directly with the coach of the team or squad when working with an athlete or group of athletes locally. I could pick up the phone and spend 5 minutes asking questions or clarifying the overall plan. Now, everything had to be done via the 'Lead.'

The first thing that a new 'lead' would ask for was 'an annual periodized plan'. They wanted me to show what all my sessions would look like a year in advance (the second thing they asked for was some 'objective testing data').

I produced a nice plan with blocks and curves on it twice for two different NGBs. I soon realised, as anyone who works in a megalithic organisation, that no one reads this stuff, especially not the Head Coach. Middle managers everywhere have to produce reports to senior managers to justify their existence. Not once in my coaching life has a Head Coach asked to see my 'annual periodized plan.

The years rolled on and every time a new 'lead' was appointed, I would get asked for the same two pieces of information. I could have cut and pasted from different sports and sent the information away but I couldn't live with myself.

I counter-punched by asking for the team schedule and sports training plans first, to 'help me plan better.' Surely if we are trying to be scientific we should analyse all the information and data before writing our plan. This failed because I never got that information back: the coaches never planned like that.

As I was learning and evolving as a coach and realising the futility of trying to predict the future, a new fresh-faced 'lead' would be appointed and I would roll over like Bill Murray to switch the clock radio off as I listened to Sonny and Cher for the umpteenth time.

"Plans are worthless, planning is everything."

General Eisenhower quoted an old Army adage when recounting his experiences organising the D-Day landings.

I now have an overall plan of key lifts and loading and progressions when to go faster or heavier and when to go lighter according to the schedule and season of our athletes. I plan in detail from week to week with sets and reps and adjustments of warm-up exercises and assistance exercises referring to the overall plan and also to my reflections and the athletes from the previous week.

And yet I still have to make adjustments in almost every session that I coach. People come in tired or late or stressed or aching or injured from life. I would be negligent if I imposed my plan on people who were unfit or unready for it.

There is nothing sacrosanct about my plans but the health and well-being of the athletes that I coach are inviolable.

37: SORE OR INJURED?

There is a difference between playing when you are injured and playing when you are sore. Both may be painful, but playing with an injury is likely to make that injury worse and take longer to heal. For the young athlete, learning to identify the difference is an essential part of their sporting journey. Every athlete will be sore at some point, many will suffer an injury.

In January 2017, Green Bay Packers receiver, Jordy Nelson, played with two broken ribs and caught six passes in the NFC Conference Championship. He was an adult, had full medical supervision, wore body armour and knew that if he played it would help his team win (they lost against the Atlanta Falcons). He knew that he would have the entire off-season to heal and get better.

Telling a 9-year-old to play through such an injury is irresponsible and should not happen. Their health and well being is more important than any sports match at their level.

What is an injury?

According to the International Olympic Committee (IOC) manual of sports injuries (2012) a sports injury may be defined as, ***"Damage to the tissues of the body that occurs as a result of sport or exercise."***

This includes everything from a blister on the palm of a weightlifter to the fractured spine of an alpine skier. The IOC definition could be extended to almost all physical training that causes an improvement in fitness: the normal overload and recovery cycle that takes place to allow the muscular, vascular and respiratory systems to adapt to the new workload.

But that does not help us define an injury.

My son's shins are covered in bruises: not from his football training, gymnastics or athletics. They are from his playground games at lunchtime. They must have hurt but he gets back into the mix. He decides to do that.

Tender Loving Care: TLC.

A 10-year old gymnast that I coach cut his heel in training this week. There was a tiny amount of blood. We took him out of training, put a plaster on it, asked if he was okay, and he went back on the mat. He sustained a sports-injury in training and carried on.

Another girl was out of breath, said her tummy was aching after rolling and wanted to stop. I asked, *"Is it sore or just tired?"*

"Just tired," she said. She sipped some water and got back on the mat.

In neither case did I ignore the athlete, nor force them to go back into training. However, we want them to be able to train when tired and get used to some fatigue so that they adapt and get fitter.

The girl could have strained a muscle, the boy could have sustained a fracture underneath the cut: as coaches, we can not pretend to know what the injury is. If the child is in distress, we need to let them sit out.

Bumps and bruises happen all the time in sport, and children need to be able to take a moment out before resuming their play. This 'time-out' will allow them to compose themselves and see if they are hurt, or just temporarily sore. A little bit of TLC with an assistant or parent-helper goes a long way to making them feel better.

Time to stop.

I have seen three boys fracture their wrists when vaulting. All about 11 years old and going through growth spurts. Each time they tried to carry on and I had to pull them out. I didn't know they had fractures at the time, they just said their arm hurt. I could see by the way that they held it that something was wrong. Tough kids who wanted to carry on, but I pulled them out before they did further harm.

If continuing training is likely to cause further harm or damage then it is time to stop, or do an alternative activity (if appropriate). Even a blister can be very painful as anyone who has had one on their heel and tried to walk will know. Carrying on in a soccer match could cause further skin damage and then the child will be unable, or unwilling, to play in the next match.

Children who complain about sore shins should be taken out of the training: stress fractures are common and are linked to overuse. In an athletics club, that child could try a throwing event for the next few sessions and then gradually return to running. That is a sensible precaution and keeps the child active and involved. If the shins are sore when throwing, then the child might have to cycle or swim: non-weight-bearing activities.

The athletics coach then might like to revisit their training programme and see how it balances with the child's other activities: they might be doing a lot in school PE or play another sport like lacrosse that has a lot of running in it. Being told to 'tough it out' on the track would be negligent in this case.

Summary.

Not all injuries require cessation of activity. Some need a short time-out, some an alternative activity, some need a day's rest. But, some require immediate medical attention. The main rule is: if carrying on is likely to cause further harm or damage then STOP.

Even if you think a child is 'faking it' there is a reason why they are doing that. TLC and giving an option to carry on is a good place to start. The coach shows empathy and compassion and the athlete will respond accordingly.

38: A 5-STEP PLAN TO CURE INSOMNIA

"Tired nature's sweet restorer," is how Shakespeare once described sleep. However, one-third of the population suffers from insomnia and rarely feels restored. Insomnia is extremely debilitating emotionally and mentally and affects motivation to train. It is different from being tired due to a short-term lack of sleep where a few lifestyle changes can improve the situation.

Insomnia can lead to a cycle of decline where motivation decreases and unhealthy habits creep in. The good news is this can be halted. Coaches and teachers need to recognise the signs in their athletes and how they will impede any performance.

Telling your athlete to 'sleep more,' is unhelpful and can exacerbate the problem.

What is insomnia?

Insomnia can be defined as any difficulty falling asleep, poor quality sleep, staying asleep or a combination of all three. This is different from just being tired due to lack of sleep. Although many of the population may be sleep deprived due to lifestyle, that can usually be rectified by going to bed earlier, or often by having 'lie-ins' at the weekend.

Sleep is a varied pattern of different states ranging from deep sleep earlier on at night, to lighter sleep nearer waking time. Waking up happens frequently but normal sleepers fall back to sleep in seconds and are unlikely to remember it. However, insomniacs often wake up and stay awake.

The onset of insomnia can be caused by many things including:

Illness
Stress
Pain
Depression
Medication
Lifestyle
Poor sleep habits

If your sleep habits and lifestyle are good, then it may be that a temporary stressful situation just leads to short-term sleep disruption. But, if the habits are bad then once the initial cause of poor sleep is removed, the insomnia remains. This then leads to a cycle of insomnia from bad habits to insomnia to more bad habits.

For example, if you have had a run of 3-4 nights of broken sleep you will be feeling what I can best describe as 'groggy' during the day. To cope with the daily demands of life, you may reach for caffeine, sugary snacks or take a nap. Or, to help you get to sleep you might reach for a nightcap. Whilst these do temporarily give you a boost (or relaxant in the case of alcohol) they can then lead to worse sleep the following night.

When this continues into weeks, months or even years, the serial insomniac views going to bed differently from that of a normal sleeper. Instead of looking forward to a good night's sleep, they go to bed hardly expecting to feel refreshed the next morning. If they wake up, then it fulfils their negative expectations and they become more anxious.

It often comes down to 'If I sleep well, I will feel good, if I sleep badly I will feel awful.' It is hard for non-insomniacs to understand how demoralising this can be.

Does insomnia affect performance?

'So what?' you may ask, 'Just get on with it' you may say, but insomnia can affect performance in many ways. To clarify again, insomnia is different from just getting a bad night's sleep occasionally which all athletes will do.

It is hard to find studies on insomnia in athletes; almost all studies only mention sleep duration or sleep quality and are short-term. One study found that elite athletes spent 8.5 hours in bed, but only slept for 7 hours a sleep efficiency rating of 81% (1). Non athletes in the same study spent 8 hours in bed but slept for 7.25 hours a sleep efficiency of 89%. Some of the elite athletes may well be insomniacs, but this wasn't diagnosed.

In another study on Australian athletes, the individual sports athletes only averaged 6.5 hours of sleep a night with the team sports players averaging 7 hours (2). However, the athletes averaged 8.4 hours in bed, with a sleep efficiency of 86%.

Swimmers and their early morning starts can suffer from 'Training jet lag' where they might only get 5.4 hours on training days and then 7.1 hours on rest days (3). Worse still, the sleep efficiency was only 71% and 77% respectively with time in bed being 7.7 hours and 9.3 hours. This is plenty of time in bed, but very inefficient. Just spending more time in bed is unlikely to help these athletes, they need to improve their sleep efficiency first.

One direct consequence of lack of sleep can be an increased likelihood of injury with adolescents sleeping more than 8 hours having a 68% reduction in chance of injury compared to those who sleep less than 8 hours (5).

In the general population, sleep deprivation is associated with a higher body mass index but whether it is a cause or an effect is hard to prove (6). Sleep deprivation can lead to a lack of motivation to train and therefore sedentary behaviour. Conversely, a lack of physical activity could lead to poor sleep quality!

One thing that is affected is your ability to think clearly because chronic sleep deprivation leads to cellular disorganization and degeneration in selected brain areas – the hippocampus, prefrontal cortex, amygdala, and hypothalamus (7). The good news is that this can be recovered with 2 good nights' sleep.

Case study.

Richard a 46 year old middle distance runner had suffered from insomnia for as long as he could remember. He had measured his sleep duration in his training diary for over 20 years and rarely had 7 hours of unbroken sleep. He got 8 hours of continuous sleep maybe once a year. Most nights he went to bed at 1030 and set his alarm for 6 am to get a good start. He is married with 2 Primary school-age children, so wanted to exercise before they got up and he went to work.

His sleep diary showed that he would get 2-3 hours of sleep, wake up for 1-2 hours and then get another 2-3 hours of lower-quality sleep before his alarm went off. If he had been awake in the night, he would often hit the snooze button and then miss training. He would then feel guilty and try to fit in more training the next day if he slept well.

As the day wore on he would reach for sugary snacks to keep going as he felt like nodding off mid-afternoon. If he worked from home he would nap after lunch to avoid the snacks. At night, if he sat down after 8 pm he would nod off. The only way to stay awake was to keep moving.

Richard had previously seen an NLP practitioner who gave him an audio tape with a series of relaxing exercises. This worked when he used it, but since being married and sharing a bed he didn't as it annoyed his wife who always went to bed first and slept soundly for 9 hours.

He finally went to see his GP about it after a friend suggested he seek help. It wasn't the lack of sleep that bothered Richard, it was his reaching for sugar, skipping exercise and then drinking wine at night to get to sleep.

The GP was sympathetic and referred him to two different appointments with specialists, one a neurologist who asked him to perform various simple motor skills, another who just said he was a hypochondriac! A year after he first saw the GP he got an appointment with a sleep clinic.

The sleep clinic consisted of 4 appointments with a sleep specialist who gave Richard information about insomnia, healthy sleep and tasks to do every week. Within 6 weeks Richard was sleeping solidly every night and a year later had had only 3 disrupted sleep nights. This is compared to having 3-4 disrupted sleep nights every week previously.

The hardest thing to do was being disciplined on the action points for the first 2-3 weeks whilst feeling extremely fatigued. However, the weekly sessions were useful as they were shared with another insomniac who was equally as distraught. Richard was able to share his thoughts freely and find out that they were typical of insomniacs, rather than feeling abnormal and trying to get 8 hours of sleep every night.

The strategies listed in this article were used, but the most effective for Richard was the sleep efficiency diary. He realised that he only needed 6 hours of sleep a night and had been trying to have much more. Rather than go to bed earlier, he got up earlier: 5 am to start with and then once established, 0515.

By being consistent with his wake-up time and working back from there he was able to sleep throughout the night. Richard decided to get up earlier rather than stay up later because he was able to be more productive in the morning.

"All I do if I stay up late is watch TV, but getting up early means I can read and then train and be ready for when the kids wake up at 7. I didn't want to be one of those weirdos who gets up at 5, but I am and feel much better for it."

A step-by-step guide to breaking the insomnia cycle.

This assumes that you have covered the basics such as avoiding screen time in the evenings, no caffeine after 3 pm and eating earlier where possible.

Step 1: Set up your bedroom for sleep.

Your bedroom is for sleeping only (and sex) so remove any obstacles or distractions to that effect. This includes books, whilst it is often advised to read before bed, you need to establish the bedroom as a place to sleep only. Read elsewhere until your eyes are shutting and then go into your bedroom.

This may involve some Marital discussions, especially if your spouse likes watching TV, checking their emails or doing their ironing when in the bedroom (and then annoyingly sleeps for 8 hours solid)!

Step 2: Reframe the insomnia as a problem to solve, rather than a reason for slipping into bad habits.

Insomniacs tend to have 2 states: awful and good. But, try to use a scale of 1-10 when you wake up in the morning with 1 being awful and 10 being excellent. You will often wake up in the range of 2-4.

Ask yourself then if eating sugary foods, avoiding easy exercise or avoiding spending time with a friend will make you feel better at the end of the day.

The answer is no and over time good habits will help improve your sleep.

Step 3: Establish a sleep schedule.

This is the hard bit. First, look at what time is the earliest you need to get up in the week and then get up at that time every day, including the weekends. If you have to get up early on Wednesday at 6 am to drive to a meeting, then that is the time you need to get up the rest of the week too. You must be disciplined in this and then your body will adjust.

Then, monitor your sleep efficiency over the next week. You do this by measuring total sleep time and average time in bed, then dividing sleep time by time in bed and multiplying by 100.

Time in bed: 480 minutes. Time asleep 360 minutes.

Sleep efficiency = (360/ 480) x100 = 75%

In this example, actual sleep time was only 6 hours, so set your bedtime for 6 hours ahead of your wake-up time. Only go to bed at this time and not before. If you are unable to sleep within 15 minutes of your new bedtime, get up and do something else outside of the bedroom.

Monitor this for a week and see what your average sleep time was and your sleep efficiency. Your sleep efficiency needs to be above 90% regularly before you extend your time in bed. Then extend it by 15 minutes and repeat the above exercise. If it is below 85% you need to reduce the time spent in bed by 15 minutes and try again.

Step 4: Set up a buffer zone.

By now you should be feeling very tired and sleeping more solidly with less time in bed. However, this is unsustainable and it is time to get better habits. One of these is a buffer zone between daily activity and sleep. This means switching off from work and domestic duties as well as not thinking about training.

For example, if you are planning to go to sleep at 11 pm, this now also means going to bed at 11 pm. The length of the buffer zone depends on what else you have to do, there is no point saying it should be 2 hours if you don't get home from training until 10 pm! But, at least 30 minutes before you plan to go to sleep you should have stopped being busy mentally.

This means switching off emails, texts and all social media. Watching TV is fine, as long as it is calming rather than stimulating. Simple things like cleaning your teeth just before bed can wake you up a bit, so try and do that earlier, as well as any other chores such as packing your training bag, or making your lunch for the next day.

If your mind is racing, try writing down the things that need to be done the next day as well as the things that are concerning you. Then write down the positive things that have happened to you that day, or that you have done, as well as something to look forward to the next day. That way you are finishing on a good note before you start your buffer zone.

This may include reading (out of the bedroom) some chores or listening to music for example. If you have a longer buffer zone, you may well start to fall asleep too early and take impromptu naps that are stealing from your night's sleep. Then you may have to do something physical to stay awake such as stretching, having a shower or going for a walk around the block.

Step 5: Stop tossing and turning.

Insomniacs will often toss and turn in frustration and being awake in bed. If you are either unable to fall asleep within 15 minutes of going to bed or are awake for more than 15 minutes in the night: get up out of bed and do something else. This will not improve your sleep that night, but it will help you sleep the next night.

Use the time to do something that you like: an extra 15 minutes of reading time or doodling or a jigsaw. You could try progressive muscular relaxation if your body is particularly tense.

Thinking about losing sleep ahead of your 'big day' only makes things worse.

When you start to nod off, go back to bed and start again. It will be tempting to hit the snooze button when your alarm goes off, but you must keep to the same wake up time.

Summary.

Being an insomniac can be downright miserable, and whilst it is unlikely to damage your health directly, it does lead to a lack of motivation and a potential uptake of bad habits. The idea that you need to get 8-9 hours' sleep per night which is often mentioned is incorrect for many people. By following the steps outlined here, you have a great chance of curing your insomnia and enjoying many good (albeit shorter) nights' sleep.

References.

1. Journal of Sports Science 30 (6) p541-545 (2012).

2. European Journal of Sports Science 14 p123-130 (2014).

3. European Journal of Sport Science, 14 (1) p310-315 (2014).

4. Biological Rhythm Research 46 (4) p523-536 (2015).

5. Journal of Pediatric Orthopaedics 34 (2) p129-133 (2014).

6. Journal of Physical Activity and Health 12 p1567-1575 (2015).

7. Biological Rhythm Research 47 (3) p425-437 (2016).

39: THE QUEST FOR ULTRA PERFORMANCE

"Each man delights in the work that suits him best."
Homer, The Odyssey.

Odysseus had his 10-year journey home to Ithaca, Jason his search for the Golden Fleece, Percival his Grail Quest and Frodo had to destroy the One Ring.

All these Heroes had to:

Travel long distances

Enlist the help of allies

Defeat enemies

Overcome obstacles

Make many sacrifices

Does this sound familiar in your training or coaching?

(Female quests are under-represented in literature: Dorothy trying to return to Kansas is a rare example.)

"If you give them silk pyjamas, they won't get out of bed."
Rob Gibson, Rugby Coach.

Whilst these Heroes had a destination in mind, the journey, the struggle, and the life-changing process were the real story. (I always question why Frodo walked when he could have hitched a ride on an Eagle).

As an athlete, having things laid out on a plate for you may not always be the best thing. Giving players underfloor heating in a changing room may be nice, but what happens when they have to play away?

"Talent needs trauma," by Dave Collins is an excellent piece on why obstacles and hazards are needed as part of Long Term Athlete Development (LTAD).

I see athletes I have worked with moving to 'Institutes' and becoming Institutionalised: they start moaning if they have to fill their water bottles, the wrong music is played in the gym, or if they have to wait for an hour in between training sessions!

A similar problem occurs with coaches who want to gain experience at a 'bells and whistles' facility. They become fascinated by the kit and use that first, rather than thinking about the athlete and the process.

Put them in an empty room with 30 kids and say *"Get them fit,"* and they turn round and ask *"Where's the force platform?"*

Earn the Right.

I have a philosophy of coaching that the athlete has to **'Earn the Right.'** I can show them the way, but they have to take the steps. Rather than turn up to our Athletic Development Club and get some fancy stash, they have to start working and assessing their ability.

Young rugby players ask, *"When are we going to do cleans?"*

I answer, *"You have to earn the right,"* which means being able to move well and efficiently first. Can they do a single-leg squat? Can they do 50 Hindu press-ups and 100 Hindu squats? Can they do a dumbbell complex first? Can they overhead squat 50% of their body weight?

It is easy to get popular in the short term by giving away kit and jumping on the latest training bandwagon.

Will that approach help the athlete when they are face down in the mud on a cold December night with a hairy-arsed monster stamping on them? Will it help them as they try and apply that power in the open field?

The same applies to coaches, you have to 'Earn the Right' to work with athletes: at any level! 6-year-old kids deserve the same amount of planning and preparation as an Olympian.

Someone said to me this week that they couldn't use their knowledge and techniques on kids that age. I said he had to *"Earn the right"* to work with those kids by improving his knowledge and learning different techniques.

Ultra Performance.

Feedback from a recent speed workshop with coaches included, *"I reckon that you are a hard taskmaster."* Perhaps, but I was emphasising the quality of execution and precision of movement before progressing.

The Quest for Ultra Performance is about the journey, the struggle and the process for coaches and athletes alike. There are no shortcuts.

"It is a mistake to look too far ahead. Only one link of the chain of destiny can be handled at a time." Winston Churchill.

We can learn from other people: mentors, senior coaches and fellow athletes to help us along the way: we then have to practice implementing that information.

We can enlist the support of allies (parents, friends, coaches, teachers): we then have to step onto the pitch, mat or court ourselves and have a go.

We can attend conferences, workshops and courses that help accelerate our learning: we then have to Plan, Do and Review. It is called the Coaching Process rather than the Coaching Destination!

No one can input the passion and desire though, the opening quote from Homer is important to understand as an athlete or coach.

The only way we can attain Ultra Performance is by undergoing the Quest.

(Thanks to Rob Frost for the Headline).

40: PLAY, PLAY AND PLAY

"How can I motivate my child to do more exercise?" Parents often ask me.

"Play with them," is my answer. This may seem simplistic but it works.

Children, up until their teenage years anyway, enjoy spending time with their parents: provided the parent is present mentally and emotionally, as well as physically.

Here are three tips on how to inspire your children to exercise so that they look forward to being healthy and active.

Tip 1: Switch off your smartphone.

If you are out in the yard or park with your child and dealing with work emails or sharing pictures on social media, then you are physically present but emotionally absent. Your child knows this. Fifteen minutes of quality play and attention will make the trip outside fun and rewarding; they will want to go back again.

Tip 2: Have a variety of sporting toys to play with.

The environment is crucial when encouraging children to play. It doesn't require a lot of money either. Here are some essentials: Soft balls of different shapes and sizes for smaller hands to throw and catch (rolled-up socks work too); skipping rope (one for parents too); a wheeled vehicle to help them keep up on walks (scooter, balance bike, skateboard); different bats/ racquets to strike with.

Or, you can roll up a magazine and tape it tight and have your child throw a screwed-up piece of paper at you. That is your indoor softball game. Their coordination needs to develop so balloons are great for them to practice (and ornament friendly).

If your child has lots of playtime with these homemade items, they develop skills that give them confidence when they are then asked to do more organised activities at school.

Children learn by watching and then doing. They will perform the activity for a short time and then want to move on to something different. This is perfectly suited for the home environment. It is less suited for an hour of adult-led coaching, especially at a young age. Fifteen minutes of play and then they can do reading, crafts or help you do the housework!

Tip 3: Train with your child rather than them training with you.

The keen endurance sports parent can be seen taking their child for runs and bike rides. Worse, they drag them along to their weekly jog in the park and force them to run slowly alongside. The child will comply because they want to spend time with Mum and Dad but you risk them dropping out completely when they get older.

(Even worse the parent counts their child's 'steps' and tells other parents how many they've done. UGH!)

Children play more like sprinters: they perform short bursts of activity and then take a rest. No child goes to the park to play with their friends and run laps. If you devote some of your training time to playing with your child on their terms, you can develop your speed and agility with them.

Here are some ideas that could help add some freshness to your training, but more importantly, help your child develop their fitness in a way appropriate to their age and stage of development.

Play ideas.

During the COVID lockdown, our Willand P.E. project had play as one-third of the lessons (the other two strands were strength and movement). You can see a simple example here (https://rb.gy/jyackb).

Fetch: A good opportunity for you to combine throwing with your child. Get any throwing object like a tennis ball or frisbee and throw it as far as you can. Both of you run to the object and then the other person throws it as far as they can. Continue across the park and then return. Alternatively, one of you throws and fetches and then the other person takes their turn. The former is more continuous, the latter has the benefit of shortening the sprint distance for the less able thrower.

Tag: A surprisingly hard classic. This is what kids live for. Have some "safe" areas but set a time limit on how long they can spend there. A smaller space means more short sprints, but more agility. A larger space means longer sprints and adults get the advantage.

Crawling: Working on reciprocal arm and leg action, hip and shoulder strength and coordination. You can either crawl for 5- 10 metres and then get up and run, which works on acceleration, or you can crawl in as many different ways as possible in a smaller space. For example forwards, backwards, sideways, hips up, hips down, on 1 hand/2legs or 2 hands/1 leg. You can either race or match what your child is doing.

With these three ideas in place, you will hopefully have fun, bond with your child, and inspire them to move more often.

They are also fundamental skills that will help them when they start any sport.

41: BEWARE THE VOLUME TRAP

"How many miles should I run?"

This is the question that endurance coach Steve Magness gets asked the most when presenting at workshops. His seminar at GAIN in 2017 covered volume and other training parameters that apply to many different sports.

I met Steve five years earlier and picked his brains at every GAIN until they fell out of his ears. I use many of his principles with our athletes, with great results. Until I met him, much of the endurance coaching I had seen or read was very patchy and full of mystical secrets or folklore.

"There is no difference between 99 miles and 100 miles, but people want to get to triple digits," Magness said (and therefore earn the right to wear the hair shirt and flail themselves). The same applies to team sports with soccer players trying to run 11km in one session because someone told them that's what they do in a match.

Steve gave two main reasons for this behaviour:

It's human nature to be obsessed with volume. It's the simplest thing we can measure, so let's measure it. (If people see me out for a run, the first thing they always ask is 'How far did you go?' never 'How fast did you run?').

We have a deep NEED for classification. It's the downside to 'what gets measured gets managed.' When we are categorised and accept a label we can then defend our label. 'I'm a low mileage/high-intensity coach.' etc.

Training load calculation.

Training load is a commonly used form of measurement.

Training load = training volume x intensity But this is too simplistic. What type of load is it?

Metabolic

Biomechanical

Neural

Psychological

How about when the load is applied?

Intensity

Density

Frequency

Rest Periods

How does this relate to daily and weekly sessions?

Front Loaded

Back Loaded

How can one number express all this accurately or in a meaningful fashion?

Weekly Training Load.

Steve broke down the weekly training load of one of his runners.

90 miles per week

10.5 hours of training (I made the point that this is for good runners; recreational runners who tried to copy the miles would be on their feet for a lot longer).

76550 calories burned

25,920ml of Oxygen consumed.

Volume has become a marker for "load" and has become a surrogate for physical stress. It is assumed the training "stimulus" leads to a kind of adaptation.

Instead, we should look at how much we NEED to do to get the positive adaptation. For example in the weekly schedule above the loading on the Achilles tendon may be the weakest link and therefore limit what another athlete can do.
Common assumptions.

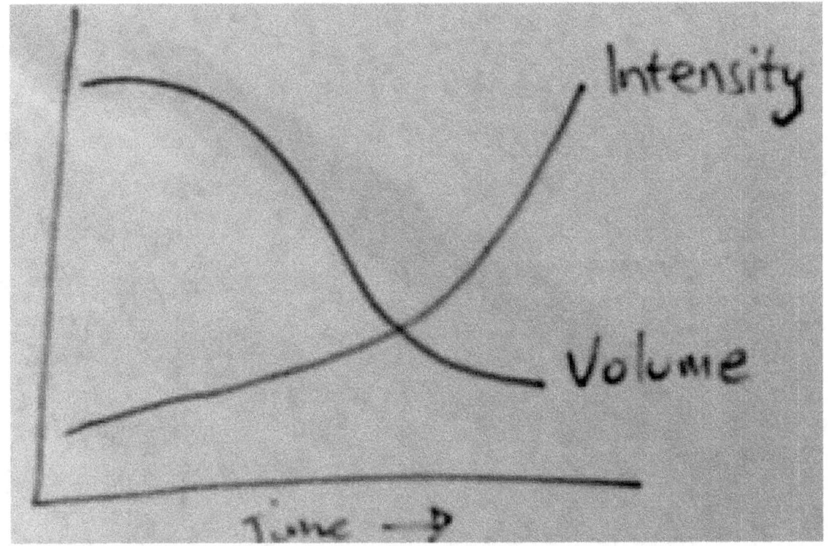

Volume vs intensity expressed simplistically

Steve gave us 3 common assumptions that may be less than certain in reality.

Assumption 1: Volume and Intensity training interact in a simplistic fashion.

Instead, there is a constant interplay that changes within each session, each week and over the longer course of a year.

Assumption 2: Volume = ONLY way of getting an aerobic adaptation.

This is simply incorrect there are many other ways of stimulating the aerobic system.
Assumption 3: Adaptation looks like this

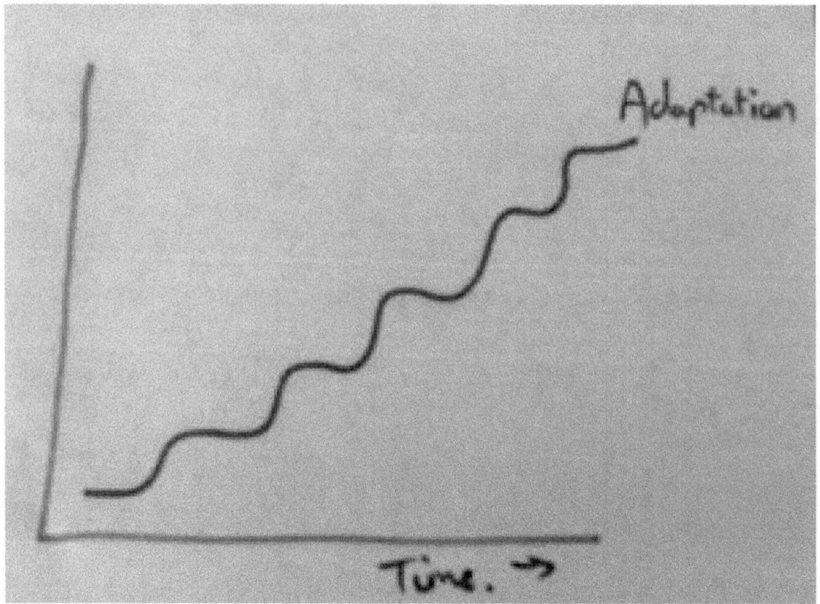

Instead, variability is the name of the game. There is a 10% rule of thumb for volume increases, but Steve gave examples from his younger self where increases were much more than this and he could adapt.

The amount of training depends on:

The athlete's perception of normal (a 120-mile-a-week runner given 90 miles would consider this light, a 50 mile a 50-mile-a-week runner may well panic!)

Physiological adaptations.

Tendon and muscle rate of adaptation: different from each other and also between athletes.

Bone Turnover (diet surely has an impact on this too?)

Steve's Old Man Strength.

Steve then gave us examples of how he could train with his athletes using his 'Old man strength' (Steve is only 32 and a middle-distance runner, I need to pull him aside the next time I see him!)

He can do the sessions thanks to an accumulated, consistent training load over time. Younger athletes can indeed increase their volume with age, after that, they can reduce it and preserve it by working on specific volumes.

Steve talked about the psychology of volume which I have found to be true depending on the athlete. Sometimes you have to adapt the programme to what the athlete feels they 'need' or at least swing the pendulum in that direction.

He then asked us to 'flip the switch' and that it was not about

Volume to get adaptation

It's thinking about

Adaptation and then how much volume is needed?

"Volume is not a master control switch."

Alternative ways of developing the aerobic system than volume.

Steve then gave some examples and case studies of how the aerobic system can be developed in middle-distance runners without just adding more weekly mileage.

Recreational runners, please take note: you do not have the time to do the mileage if you are running slower than 5-6 minute miles. If you try and copy the mileage plans of faster runners you will be spending a lot more time training than they do!

Some session examples include:

Pre-fatigue: do a shorter 'long run' the day after an intense workout.

Doubles: do 2 shorter runs in a day, helps with lifestyle too.

Strength session followed by endurance work. You are forced to train in this fatigued state.

Ending the session or cooldowns with 'stuff.' For example an 800m 'cruise' to work at the high end of the aerobic system and get used to preserving strength at the end of a race.

Steve then gave some examples of sessions which he has done with his athletes including the sets/ reps and different ideas. All of these worked with his athletes and in their context.

(I often see endurance coaches trotting out a session like 'Oregon circuits' or such and inflicting it upon their athletes year after year without understanding why. So I won't post the details here to avoid feeding the monster. I do use some of the ideas with Excelsior ADC athletes).

Measuring for measuring sake.

Steve finished his seminar with some questions about measuring sessions and how these questions can then shape what we do as coaches.

If athletes are constantly looking at technology, how can they 'feel' what they are doing? (Luke destroyed the Death Star by using the Force remember, not by looking at his Garmin).

This is even assuming you are measuring the right thing. I have written elsewhere about the addiction to measuring technology and how that can then alter the design of sessions. The tail wags the dog. Bryan Fisher summed it up a few years ago at GAIN:

"Heart rate should be an indicator, not a dictator".

Ask yourself these questions when developing a middle-distance running plan (or any other plan for that matter) for an athlete:

In what direction are we trying to adapt?

Where have they been in the past?

Are they still adapting?

What is their injury history and adaptability?

What is the risk-to-benefit ratio of your programme will it cause adaptation or maladaptation/ injury?

Are we measuring the right thing?

Is that measurement what you think it is?

Is the answer to any of these questions *'You should run X miles per week'*?

The answer isn't to be anti-volume or pro-volume, it is to sit down and think about the athlete in front of you and work out what is right for them. How many coaches take the time to do that?

Summary.

Much like when I first saw Frans Bosch present on sprinting in 2009, I had an
'Aha' moment and thought Steve's approach made sense (although Frans
didn't make any sense the first 3 times I saw him, but I could see it worked).
Steve is very good at expressing complex ideas simply.

42: THE DANGERS OF LABELLING YOUTH ATHLETES

Youth coaches pick teams to win matches at the weekends. If they win on Saturday, they are deemed to have done a good job. However, this one match is only a single step in each of the young athletes' journeys. If coaches and teachers label the athlete as 'talented', 'fast', 'lazy', 'stupid' or 'clever' then they are risking hindering the growth and development of those athletes.

Youth sports should be about fun, inclusivity and development. Youth coaches and p.e. teachers are responsible for all the athletes in their care: too many people drop out of sports as it is.

Instead of labelling children and putting them into convenient boxes, coaches should be open-minded as to the children's potential. If they give hope to everyone in the programme then all the children work and strive to become better versions of themselves.

As Finn Gunderson told me, *'Forget winning or losing. Aren't we saving souls here?'*

Some common misconceptions.

The early developer who is bigger, stronger and faster than her peers may be labelled 'talented' and then struggle to adapt when her peers catch up. She may not develop the work ethic necessary to succeed at anything long-term. Instead, she relies on her 'talent.'

The coach who wants to win on Friday picks the early developer because she is a head taller than her peers. If the coach uses the word, 'talent,' then other athletes believe themselves to be untalented. This can then result in them quitting or not trying, using phrases such as, 'I'm no good, so what's the point?'

The athlete labelled, 'lazy,' may quit the sport. The 'lazy' athlete may lack self-confidence or understanding of the sport. They may have outside pressures from home, peers or school that affect their motivation in training and be misinterpreted as 'lazy.' A coach who encourages and praises this athlete helps build their confidence.

Work ethic can be developed but it takes time. Structured practices that challenge the athletes' minds, as well as their bodies, create enthusiasm. So do semi-structured practices where the athletes teach their peers or follow the guided discovery.

The dangers of labelling.

The thought of defining any person with one or two words is mystifying. Every human is a complex individual. We have multiple attributes that include our physical, emotional, mental and social makeup. Labelling can quickly degenerate into stereotyping. Coaches and teachers can preconceive what an athlete from a certain ethnic/social/economic background will be like without seeing the athlete in action. This then leads to coaching that athlete in a certain way: drill master, sycophant, disdainful (none of which are great).

In the UK, children are put into '**Talented and Gifted**' streams at school as young as 8 years old. They are labelled as such by Primary School teachers who have had four hours of Physical Education training whilst learning to become a teacher.

What is the teacher identifying?

Those who can perform skills or who win the running, jumping and throwing events. What happens to those children? They are asked to represent the school at inter-school competitions.

The teacher does not have to teach: they just select those that can do already. What happens to the rest of the children? Those that are not members of sports clubs, do not have parents who play 'catch' in the park, or who are born in the last two months of the school year and are smaller than their classmates?

They get left behind and then left out.

This continues into secondary school where children are split into two p.e. streams: able and less able! The same selection policies occur. Half of the school intake is sidelined. Half! At 11-years old.

The school teams are selected from an ever-shallower pool of athletes. Those labelled as 'less able' at 11 years old are unlikely to rejoin the pool of habitual exercisers and sports participants. Unless a rounded physical education programme teaches them the skills and includes them in games and sports with their peers.

Does any coach or teacher want to hamper a child's life chances by labelling them at 10 or 11 years old?

Summary.

Young athletes are human beings first, sportspeople second. The coach and teacher of the young athlete should recognise that during these formative years, children are changing rapidly. They can be brilliant in one situation on one day and terrible in another situation the next day.

Whilst we all like winning on Saturday, being open-minded and creative as coaches allows us to see the potential in every young athlete. We can then invent and structure different types of challenges and competitions to allow every young athlete the chance to flourish and reach their potential. No matter how long that takes.

43: HOW TO HANDLE A LOSING STREAK

If there is one guarantee in sport, it's losing. Most seasons that have playoffs and cups will result in every team, bar one, losing their last match. Losing is a part of sport and athletes and coaches don't have to like it, but they have to accept it.

A losing streak is when a team suffers a series of losses. This can occur when a team is poor and will end in relegation or when it is average to good but loses to opponents that it might normally beat.

The team that is likely to get relegated may enjoy success in the league below. This is common in UK professional soccer and rugby leagues where the bottom two or three teams are perennial relegation/promotion contenders: too strong for the lower leagues but not quite good enough to contend at a higher, and more expensive, level.

The team that is in the right league, but suffering a losing streak, can do something to halt the slide. Fortunately, unlike the movie, 'Major League', superstition and rituals are unnecessary to return to winning habits.

Don't panic.

It's easy to think that desperate times require desperate measures. Coaches think that if they have lost three games in a row then they have to make radical changes. Pressure can come from owners, fans, parents and the media. The knee-jerk reaction to external criticism can result in flawed decisions such as benching good players or changing tactics that have helped you win in the past.

The worst decision a coach can make is one that is done to silence the external voices.

This does not mean being complacent or rigidly refusing to change. It does mean taking time to reflect on what has been working as well as what could be improved.

The coach and players must have time alone and space to think. Tired and stressed personnel rarely make good decisions.

Set aside thirty minutes of non-screen, non-phone time, every day to allow yourself time to recharge and reflect. Having young children is a wonderful distraction from the madness of sports: they force you to focus on their needs right now. Walking your dog, phoning an elderly relative (who is not a sports fan) or cooking a meal with your partner are good breaks.

Reflect.

Now that your head is momentarily clear. Ask:

What has worked in the past?

What is still working?

What can be improved?

Are the opponents better, or were our tactics wrong?

Did the players execute well under pressure?

Is there a common theme between the losses?

Are your practices helping you translate ideas into action or are they simply busy work that does not help improve performance?

Ask for input from assistant coaches and players. It is common for coaches under pressure to become more isolated and more autocratic.

But the coach can not win the match. Only the players can.

It is not a sign of weakness to ask for ideas, it is a sign of confidence in your ability to harness the potential of your team. The players and assistant coaches see things from a different perspective than you do. An open forum with the whole team is difficult to manage and can get out of hand. You can get players to answer a couple of questions to start things in small groups and this often leads to freer discussions.

Three questions that I ask are:

1.   'What was the best minute of play we have had in the last two matches?'

2.   'What helps you play your best?

3.   'What part of the tactics could we practice more?'

The first question reminds the players that they do some things well and can play well.

The second gives me an insight into their motivation and how we can help bring out their best.

The third also lets me know where I might fail in communication or practice design. All of these are non-threatening and non-judgemental. They are giving the players a chance to be involved and to give me valuable information.

Be constructive.

Throwing extra laps and punishment workouts at players only serves to alienate and reinforce an 'us versus them' culture within the team. That might look good in the movies but rarely works in real life unless you have a large squad with talented and compliant reserves.

Instead, think of changing things for the better. Change the warm-up routine in practices to incorporate some fundamental work on catching, passing, and agility. Put a small, fun, game in at the end so that players remind themselves how to 'play.' Add a teaching session on the field or on the whiteboard to ensure everyone understands why you use certain tactics and then how to use them. Put the new tactic into an opposed game in practice so the players get to apply it. Ask them for feedback, listen to their suggestions, and use them!

One way to show that you have listened is to put up a graphic of ideas that have come from players and what you have done. It might be changing a pre or post-game meal, the half-time drinks, or even the music played on the team bus.

It is important to block out the external noise, especially social media, and to bond as a team. If the players are playing together and understand why your tactics are in place and how they can use them, you are off to a good start. Showing highlights of good plays from every match is also important rather than just criticising the mistakes (this needs to be done but with a solution and not in a public humiliation).

Winning is not guaranteed, the other team want to win too, but you can put good systems and habits in place and work together to give you the best chance possible.

If all else fails, you can start putting on your left shoes first and avoid walking under ladders.

44: THE OXYMORONIC TALENT PATHWAY

If you read biographies of a previous generation of sporting superstars there is usually a mention of a dedicated p.e. teacher or coach at a local sports club. Children discovered their love for the sport locally and affordably. They might have had a keen parent, like Tim Henman or Seb Coe, but most stumbled into the sport through normal p.e. and games or by going with a friend to a local club.

The sport was fun and well-coached and this led to some successes and a desire to do a bit more training. There were no academies or pathways.

'Sport for all' was the Sport England motto.

This changed with the introduction of the National Lottery and the mechanisation of sport in the UK, especially after the 'failure' of Team GB at the Atlanta Olympics. Medal tables and podium places took the place of 'Sport for all.'

Funding was dependent on National Governing Bodies (NGBs) meeting top-down objectives, including having a 'pathway' despite there being no evidence of such a thing working in reality. In his book, 'The Talent Lab,' Owen Slot summarises the report into Britain's subsequent (and expensive) pursuit and attainment of medals thus,

'There is no one single element of success, no one cap that fits all.'

The goal of UK sport was to win more Olympic medals and that was achieved: between the Atlanta Games and Rio (2016), GB won 96 medals.

However, just 12 people won or contributed to 49 of them.

Over half the medals were won by just a dozen individuals.

Or, to put it another way, '*Is this a good use of public money?*'

Where is the Olympic Legacy?

In the twelve years after the London Olympics, there has been a decrease in sporting participation. Part of that can be blamed on the COVID-19 pandemic and the various lockdowns. However, the pandemic may have hastened the decline rather than caused it.

Two stark facts should be first and foremost on the minds of parents, teachers, coaches and public health figures:

1. Only 1 in 5 adolescents and adults meet the current weekly recommendations for aerobic and muscle-strengthening exercises for health across 31 countries.

2. The reported levels of anxiety and depression in adolescent athletes in the USA are higher now than they were pre-Covid.

In other words, 80% of adolescents are not doing enough exercise to stay healthy.

Those that do play sports have more mental health issues than they did before Covid even though they have returned to activity.

And yet...

There are more 'talent pathway managers' than coaches in NGBs nowadays. More 'scholarships' and 'academies' and 'talent programmes' than there are minibuses to ferry the kids around. As soon as a child shows an interest (or an early growth spurt or specialisation), they are 'identified' and told they 'must' attend a training/ selection camp miles away from home.

Those working within 'Talent Pathways' operate in an echo chamber where they attend conferences with other people in similar roles from different sports and share 'best practice' ideas! For those on an NGB salary, it is understandable that no one raises their hand and says,

'Hold on! Shouldn't we be focussed on helping young people get healthy and active and supporting them rather than cherry-picking from an ever-decreasing pool of participants?'

They would risk losing their job and their salary, so they stick to the company line.

Too much, too early.

NGBS are continuing to encourage young children to specialise, especially girls because they are afraid of losing 'talent' to another sport (see the Talent ID Bun Fight). They might not say so overtly, but when a child is told that they must attend weekly 'talent' sessions miles away and go to regular camps involving overnight stays, time and logistics prevent that child from doing anything else.

When I worked with England Golf, the regional (under-16 coaches) were told to:

1. Only select those girls who would definitely play for England at the senior level (!)

2. Select them at under 13 so they would 'be in the system for longer.'

These young girls had barely started secondary school and they were put into the system. They were ill-equipped physically and emotionally for this intense training and expectation. Many of them quit the sport or just returned to their home coaches and courses.

The perverseness of the NGB means that the child is in danger of dropping out of all sports: burnout, injury, or competing demands such as schoolwork are the major causes.

The increased cost of fuel and a squeeze on family incomes means that even fewer children can afford to travel big distances, let alone afford overnight stays, to play sports.

And, it is worth repeating, there is no evidence that early selection at a young age leads to representation at a senior level: in fact, the opposite is often the case.

In German football, those playing in the National Team specialised later and played more 'pick-up' games with their friends than those just playing in the Bundesliga. The players who specialised earliest and had less 'free-play' ended up playing in semi-professional teams below the Bundesliga.

At some point, specialisation and more investment in training will be necessary: but it is at a later age than you think and only when the child is ready. Playing a variety of sports, locally, with friends still works at a young age.

If they are still sleeping with a teddy bear they should not be specialising.

Questions for parents to ask.

Parents are bombarded with information from NGBs and often told that their child 'has' to be on the pathway to be successful. I suggest that parents ask the NGB the following questions:

1. Why?

2. Is there evidence that these 'pathways' work?

3. Can my child be successful without attending this academy?

4. Did any of the elite performers in your sport use a different route?

5. How much will it cost?

6. What happens if they are de-selected: will you help support them back at their club?

The answers that could be given are:

1. To show that the NGB is 'doing something.'

2. Yes: for some people but not for all (as does every method). And there is a recency bias.

3. Yes: if given the right support and encouragement locally.

4. Yes, of course, they did. Some didn't even start the sport until their late teens.

5. A lot: fuel, time, accommodation. Money that could be best spent elsewhere (unless you are wealthy).

6. No. The risk of dropping out entirely is high because the child perceives themselves as a 'failure' if they do not make the next set of teams.

Excelsior Athletic Development Club.

Our club philosophy is to help every athlete get better. It is not to produce champions nor is it to be part of a 'pathway.' Every person has different motivations for training including:

· Goal/success driven

· Feeling fit and good about themselves.

· Looking good

· Hanging out with friends

· Learning a new skill.

All of these are valid and worthwhile. The problems only occur when there is a mismatch between their motivations for training and their willingness to train enough or if the coach's expectations don't match the athlete's.

A goal-driven athlete who doesn't want to train frequently will be frustrated when they fail to meet their goals.

The athlete who wants to feel fit and hang out with friends will be frustrated/upset if the coach (me) tries to make them compete.

This comes down to communication and education. If our athletes can meet their expectations at our club they will continue to participate and see the benefits. This is led by them and facilitated by the coach.

It is not driven by an NGB setting targets.

We coach people at our club, not statistics. It is worthwhile remembering the old motto, 'Sport for All,' and helping the young generation along their journeys of discovery rather than forcing them onto someone else's pathway.

45: THE THREE STAGES OF FITNESS TESTING

'I test athletes to justify my job,' is one reason that fitness testing has become maligned and dreaded by coaches and athletes alike.

Others include: *'To look professional,' 'To use my new bit of kit,'* or *'To identify talent.'*

None of these should be reasons to waste athletes' valuable time and energy. Inaccurate, irrelevant and ill-informed tests are a sure-fire way to lose respect and credibility.

Just because your athletes don't have a choice (P.E. teachers/ college lecturers/ NGB staff) doesn't mean you should go through the motions. When advising teams and athletes on fitness tests, I make sure we discuss three things:

1.   Choosing the right test.
2.   Testing accurately and reliably.
3.   Analysing and giving feedback.

If the coach/organisation can not explain how the three points will work to the athletes, I suggest they don't bother.

Choosing the right test.

Do we need to test? Is it more measurement and monitoring rather than 'testing'? This is the first discussion point. My default position is Monitor rather than Test. I need a good reason to test and it could be:

•   To see if what we are doing is working.

•   To measure progress.

•   To evaluate the players so that we can cluster them for training.

We set off by dividing the tests into health, general and specific. Health tests include biomarkers that could be considered as monitoring or measurement. Height, weight, sleep, mood, skinfolds, heart rate, and the sympathetic nervous system can all be monitored regularly with little effort, just consistency.

Some physical competency could also be included in this category. An overhead squat or single-leg squat could be included in every warm-up and observed.

General tests would give us information about the specific fitness parameter being trained. These might include most strength tests, field endurance tests, agility and speed tests.

We know how good our athletes are at performing these tests. Again, we are measuring what the athletes are doing in training, so we could conduct this in our training sessions.

Specific tests would be relevant to the sport and replicate specific actions: The tennis fan drills, countermovement jumps or medicine ball throws, and the rugby union endurance test that requires down and up movements.

These tests should be able to isolate one component of performance that is extremely applicable to that sport.

Agility tests that last 30 seconds, treadmill incremental VO2 max tests for Judoka, and shuttle runs for 800m runners are examples of tests that either measure more than one thing or are the wrong test for that athlete.

Measuring accurately and reliably.

One of my pet hates (there are many) is watching athletes get inaccurately tested by 'pseudoscientists.' Athletes want to get the best scores, so will find ways to cheat and take shortcuts. This might be stopping 2cms short of each line on the yo-yo test, or going over cones rather than around them.

To make the test reliable, strict warm-up protocols need to be observed, as does the order of testing. If you change the warm-up before each testing day or change the order of tests, then they are unreliable. The data becomes invalid.

Carrying spare batteries, masking tape, spare pens and a stopwatch are essential tools for the tester.

What appears to be 'common sense' or 'obvious' is often forgotten in the maelstrom of testing big groups of athletes and pressure.

The test should be able to be conducted by different testers who record the same results (inter-tester reliability). It should have a uniform surface and equipment (preferably minimal).

There is a tendency to use expensive equipment to measure simple fitness parameters: this is often led by people who sell the fancy equipment!

The Cooper test is a 12-minute endurance run, designed by Kenneth Cooper, to be conducted on a 400-metre oval track. I have seen this done around a 15-metre square on a slipper netball court, as well as in various sports halls.

Try running around a 15-metre square for 12 minutes and tell me how soon your inner leg started to scream, "STOP!"

The data gained can not be compared to external athletes who conduct it on a 400-metre track.

Analysing and giving feedback.

Another pet hate (I told you I had a few) is athletes being subjected to tests by pseudo-scientists who then go off with the data and use it for their 'research' projects. (Steve Ingham does an excellent job of explaining the pitfalls in testing athletes in his book, *'How to Support a Champion'*).

If an athlete has worked their nuts off in testing and the coach has allocated time aside for it, then the information must be analysed and shared. This must be done in a way that can be understood by all the parties concerned. I learned a lot from the data visualisation and infographics course I did 10 years ago.

Look at the difference between these two graphs:

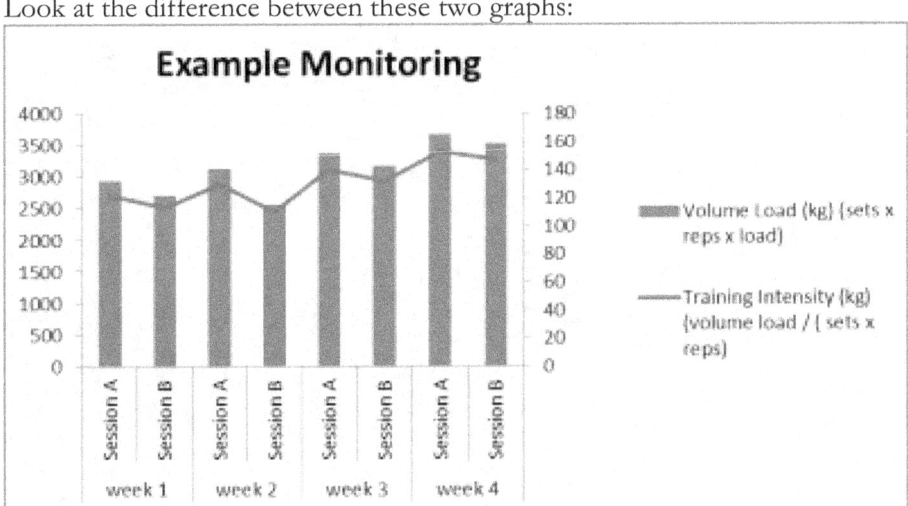

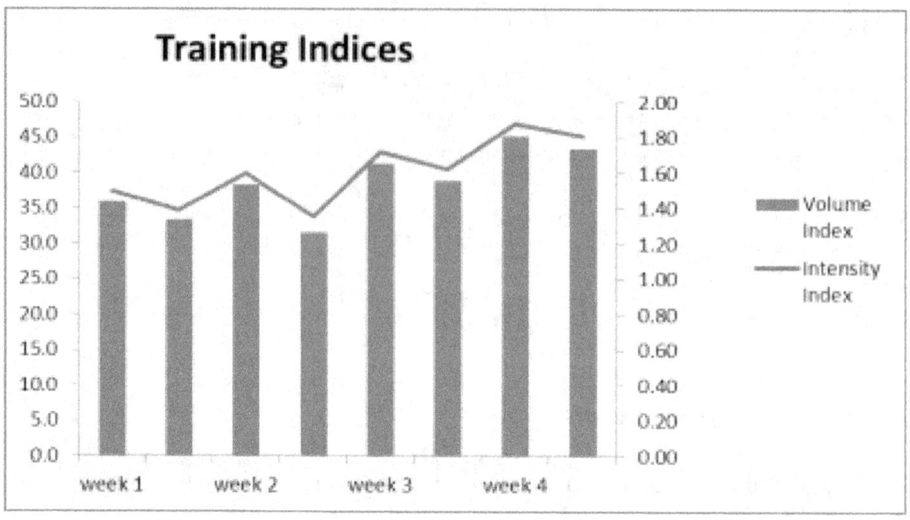

Which one is clearer?

Can you see why that is? There is less clutter in the second chart.

It is quite easy to get sucked into a trap of designing graphs and charts that look pretty in 3D colour. However, as with all aspects of coaching, it is our job to make the information as clear, relevant and understandable as possible.

Summary.

Fitness testing has its place but, just like the athletes, it has to earn its place in the schedule. If the information gained can be used to inform and change practice, then use it. If not, then don't do it. The athletes will thank you.

46: CREATING FRANKENSTEIN'S MONSTER IN THE GYM

"Man," I cried, "how ignorant art thou in thy pride of wisdom!"
— Mary Shelley, Frankenstein

I was asked last week my thoughts about using the barbell hip thrust in the gym. I had no thoughts on the matter, I don't use it as an exercise tool.

Rather than, *'What do you use to develop hip extension?'* The follow up question was, *"Why not? S&C coach X says it works on hip extension which is really important in sprints and jumps."*

Earlier that week I had been asked by a novice weight lifter why their Crossfit 'coach' was telling them different cues than I was for the snatch, especially concerning the hip extension. She prefaced this with, *"What I did with you really helped, I understood it and it works."*

Why can't we leave it at that? If what I do when I coach works, why ask me to comment on what I am NOT doing?

"Of what a strange nature is knowledge! It clings to a mind when it has once seized on it like a lichen on a rock."
— Mary Shelley, Frankenstein

Here are some exercises that I do not use, or have not used in at least 12 years:
Nordic curls
Barbell Hip Thrusts
Bench Press
The Plank

Whilst their proponents will argue their validity, I avoid simplistic isolated exercises that work on certain body parts in the hope that they will magically come together when the athlete tries to move fast or powerfully in the arena.

All of the above minimise or eliminate movement, and have a low-skill component. That makes them easier to load and develop and measure. If we can measure the exercise, we 'prove' progress.

But, expecting the isolated exercises to work together is like Frankenstein working furiously in his laboratory, and then dismayed at the result.

"*Hateful day when I received life!' I exclaimed in agony. 'Accursed creator! Why did you form a monster so hideous that even you turned from me in disgust? God, in pity, made man beautiful and alluring, after his own image; but my form is a filthy type of yours, more horrid even from the very resemblance. I am solitary and abhorred.' — The Monster*"
— Mary Shelley, Frankenstein

Whip cracking.

Last Sunday, whilst waiting for my daughter to finish horse riding, I had a go at cracking a whip. A big long one that probably weighed 200g or so. I attempted it a dozen times, and my arm was getting tired. The horse riding instructor said it looked like I was fly fishing.

I had a few more attempts and managed to crack it twice. The speed and timing were what was needed to succeed not any strength. It's embarrassing when a 60-year-old lady can do a skill faster and better than I can. I doubt if she is stronger than me at those dumbbell exercises but her timing and coordination when cracking the whip are far superior.

If I was a Frankenstein coach, I might give myself these exercises to help me get better at whip cracking:
Wrist curls
Bicep curls
Front shoulder raises

Because these are the individual components of the whip action, so surely doing these will help? This type of thinking happens all the time.

If you spend all the time in the laboratory (or weights room) without seeing, or being responsible for the end results, you can come up with all sorts of concoctions. Other mad scientists can marvel at your work and you will become famous amongst your peers.

I prefer to help our athletes get better at their chosen endeavours. This means using encouraging movement patterns that reflect the sport or use exercises that develop their speed, power and coordination. Sprinting, jumping and the snatch are coordination exercises that require practice and skill and a coach who understands them.

Beware the Frankenstein coach and the ungainly athletes who emerge from their gyms.

47: A MOVEMENT MANIFESTO

Humans have evolved through adaptation to moving in their environments. I aim to help people learn to enjoy movement and make it part of their physical and mental selves.

Coaches, teachers and parents should set an example to their athletes, students and children. This doesn't mean 'crushing' it at the gym, it means moving.

Physical activity is often reduced to a number: '10,000 steps,' 'walk a mile a day,' or '100 reps'. By focusing on the number you eliminate joy, discovery and variety. That is a quick way to put people off.

My Movement Manifesto will hopefully encourage people of all ages to participate and explore movement.

3 Mantras:

· Move well, move often.

· Variety is the spice of exercise.

· Monotony ages you, novelty invigorates you.

Locomotion: moving!

Rhythmical, continuous movements such as cycling, walking, running, swimming, skipping rope and rowing are essential for heart health and overall well-being. They form the foundation of aerobic (with oxygen) fitness and the continuous, cyclical, rhythmical action is also good for mental health and stress relief.

Other activities such as gardening, climbing and dancing are useful too but are more intermittent by their nature.

Talking of nature, doing these activities outdoors, in natural environments has proven health benefits compared to doing the same exercises indoors. Walking in parks, fields, woods and hills is different from walking on a treadmill watching TV.

Resistance Training: Overcoming Gravity.

We need resistance training to improve our bone and muscle strength. Gravity is continuously working upon us and our posture suffers. We also need strength to perform activities of daily living such as shopping, laundry and picking up children.

Resistance training includes bodyweight exercises (jumping, climbing, hanging) and the use of external resistance (dumbbells, sand disks, medicine balls, Indian clubs, barbells and kettlebells).

The use of chairs and benches to perform sitting and lying down exercises is not recommended. unless you are injured. because they restrict movement. Train your whole body: from fingernails to toenails.

The heavier the load, the less variety you can incorporate into your training. A balance of simple exercises with heavier loads and expansive exercises with lighter loads is good.

Move like a child.

Children learn to move by rolling and crawling. They love to hang from things and explore the environment. Every day is a learning day and they are delighted with every new skill.

Moving like a child will help connect your mind and body: you will be playful in attitude and purposeful when you learn new skills. Getting up and down and moving around the ground helps you coordinate and link all the parts of your body. This strengthens and stretches joints, muscles and fascia (the connective tissue under your skin) that upright activities are less able to do.

Learning new things breaks up your routine and habits. This stimulates the mind and body and forces them to adapt and become more adaptable. Learning is also fun. Try one new exercise or variation every week or work on a new skill until you are competent and then try another.

Change the speed.

Move fast, move slow, change your speed. The simpler the exercise, the easier (and safer) it is to move fast or to add some resistance. Sprinting needs to be done fast! Squats are a simple exercise that can be loaded through resistance or volume.

Forward rolls, the downward dog stretch and jumping over obstacles require different speeds but are all finite in the amount you can do.

Have some slow movements that require control and balance and stretch you.

Have some fast movements that require a greater effort and then rest.

No one mode of movement is the answer to everything.

We all have our preferences and it is great to do more of what we like. Including a little bit of everything else will help you maintain a healthy, balanced enjoyment of movement throughout your life.

If you are a runner, lift some weights and try yoga.

If you are a weight lifter, go for a long walk or a swim.

If you are a tennis player, try climbing (you have to use both arms) or learn to do a handstand.

Summary.

We are all different so following a single plan is unlikely to succeed. Our modern environments are, for the most part, safe and ordered and we easily adjust. Our movement needs to change to create change within our bodies and minds.

Move

Overcome

Learn

Change

Enjoy

48: GO HARD, GO FAST, FINISH IT, GO AGAIN

The headline quote sums up Jim Radcliffe's approach to training teams at Oregon University. I attended over a dozen of his lectures at GAIN, many of his 'Movement Madness' morning sessions and was privileged to receive some additional 1-1 tuition on his warm-up preps and hurdling technique.

His influence on my coaching and how we train athletes at our club can not be understated.

His lecture at one of my early GAINs on his training system was a masterclass on organisation. The important principle is that his workouts are efficient from beginning to end.

This was not some periodisation lecture, instead it showed the different aspects that need training, and how they connect. Radcliffe showed the different roots and branches of what is needed and why.

His lecture the previous year looked more at the weekly and monthly cycles. This looked at more of the progressions that fit into those cycles.

Musculoskeletal health 101.

Radcliffe started by linking the different aspects of fitness that are interconnected using Frank Dick's model (1984). He has changed this slightly and replaced mobility with movement efficiency and uses a pyramid analogy instead of a triangle. Radcliffe wants his players to be around as long as the pyramids have been!

He then gave his view of what physical state his college players are in when they arrive. As we all find, they have:

Poor mechanics

Poor understanding of their own body

Poor hip mobility (too much time in seated postures)

Weak torsos

Poor knee, hip and ankle integrity.

(Posture coming up time and time again).

These areas must be addressed before anything else. *"**We must be prepared to teach, train and develop not from scratch, but from behind zero.**"*

Radcliffe used a clock diagram on several of his slides asking *"What percentage of time is spent..?"*

E.g.: how much time should be spent on sitting or lying exercises that work on 1 or 2 joints or muscles in isolation compared to standing exercises that are multiple joints and require synchronisation?

*"**Running is a skill. It should be the main skill, and it needs to be taught.**"*

Poor postures, lifestyles and inadequate teaching have left the players unable to run.

The exercises and progressions in the gym should be able to assist and enhance this, rather than inhibit it. Radcliffe uses a small battery of tests/ screening exercises to assess what the players can do, rather than what they can't do.

He then leads into a progression of hip actions: Hip Hinge- Hip projection- Whip from the hip, This is done in the gym and on the field. Everything must work together.

Acceleration, Acceleration, Acceleration.

*"**Did I mention we do a lot of acceleration?**"* Radcliffe keeps working on this.

*"**Until we get better and more efficient. Otherwise, we are just running for running's sake. Get better, then repeat it.**"*

This was the central thrust of the Oregon system. Instead of doing drills for drills' sake, the coaches are asked to train skills and get them working well. This sounds a lot more like 'Coaching' rather than 'Instructing.'

(For those of you unfamiliar with College Football, Oregon was notorious for playing fast-and-furious football in the Chip Kelly ear. Other teams struggled to keep up).

Warm Up is a chance to rehearse skill.

Radcliffe espoused the use of the warm-up as a chance to rehearse skills. It should not only do the physiological things that are necessary but also be enabling skill. What you do 6 minutes before the game should build on what you did 6 hours, 6 days, 6 weeks and 6 months before.

Do you Stretch/Manipulate or do you Move before matches? (Static stretching is still commonplace in team warm-ups at College football.)

He then showed some great data on different warm-up protocols and their effect on performance. Total synchronised body lifts that moved load at speed (the snatch) helped prepare the body better than just dynamic warm-ups.

(For the younger readers, you might think '***We know this,***' but who do you think has led the field in questioning previous practices?)

Mass- Specific Force.

Are you moving mass just to move mass? Or does it have an application on the field? (We know where the UKSCA paradigm is on this!) Force ends up displaying itself on the field on one small spot like the ball of the foot, so any strength gained in the gym must be applicable.

Great force is exerted over a small base of support and rapidly. Training must replicate this and also work on the righting/ tilting reflexes that happen when the athlete is in the air or lands. Radcliffe has three main principles when training his football players:

Get 'em strong

Train Rate of Force Development

Dynamic Strength

My understanding from this lecture and the previous year is that Radcliffe incorporates application into every session, but to varying degrees. If maximal strength is being developed, at least 1-2 exercises at the end are used to help the body apply it.

Gassers vs Get-Offs.

"How much time is spent on Biomechanical Performance Technique vs Mental Toughness Training?"

In other words, is your training designed to replicate and encourage great technique and efficiency, or is it just making your players tired?

(For non-US readers a gasser is a Football conditioning drill that requires players to run 2 widths of the pitch, rest and repeat. A Get-off is working the first 2-3 steps of a start, so a 5-10 metre acceleration drill).

Radcliffe gave examples of wrestling coaches who insisted on their players doing a 13-mile run once a fortnight for "mental toughness". When you step onto the mat you want to be sure you are technically, and tactically superior, not that you can last longer on a 13-mile run (Or we may as well get Mo Farah to wrestle!).

This applies across all sports because someone has analysed the total distance covered in soccer/ basketball matches as 10km (roughly) coaches think you have to go out and jog for 10km!

What this means is that poor running mechanics are rehearsed, the over striders over stride and then hamstrings are torn when sprinting. Instead, work on the quality of the movement, then increase the reps, sets or frequency of the training. This allows the players to repeatedly produce quality work.

The same applies in the gym: Radcliffe knows his stuff works because if you ask an athlete to design their training it consists of a lot of steady-state running, bench press and bicep curls.

Because they are easy to do!

Programme Objectives (Jim Radcliffe workouts in action).

Oregon's long-term objectives are to develop:

Explosive Power

Functional Strength

Directional Speed

Transitional Agility

In the Short Term, they work on:

Power Reliability (used to call it power endurance)

Work Capacity (The ability to do more intense work, or more load, finish it, recover, go again)

Recoverability

Stamina

Radcliffe broke the Programme components down and showed how they interrelate with Preparational Work-Technical Work-Developmental Work and then Transitional Work and their various sub-divisions.

This was quite enlightening and showed the system behind the various exercises.

The Programme emphasis is to put the players in situations where the drill forces the body to learn and adapt. This is a key coaching point and shows the importance of what we do.

(As an aside, if, as an S&C coach, you just get your players to do lifts for lifts' sake and do not work with the coaches, you will get isolated and not be aiding the players get better for where it counts. You must coach.)

Summary.

Once again this session highlighted why Radcliffe is at the top of his game. He has created a system over the last 26 years that is very thorough and specific. He understands the importance of application in the game situation and knows how to get his players there.

He has researched the different aspects of power, strength, speed and agility and is continually looking to evolve his programme. This has been done with real athletes across different sports over many years.

In combination with his superb practical demonstrations, Radcliffe makes me want to improve my delivery, my planning and my thinking. I have incorporated many of his ideas into our pre-season training plans.

49: HOW TO MAKE PRE-SEASON TRAINING INTERESTING, RELEVANT AND MORE FUN

'I hate Pre-Season training.'

This is often the thought of players who are forced to undergo various fitness tests and long slow runs as part of a pre-season training and fitness programme.

Doing repeated doggies, shuttle runs and various circuits, with barely a ball in sight, is enough to put most players off.

It doesn't have to be this way.

As a Coach, you can make pre-season training interesting, relevant and more fun. Your players will be fitter, faster and stronger. More importantly, if they are willing, engaged and able to play, they will put more effort in.

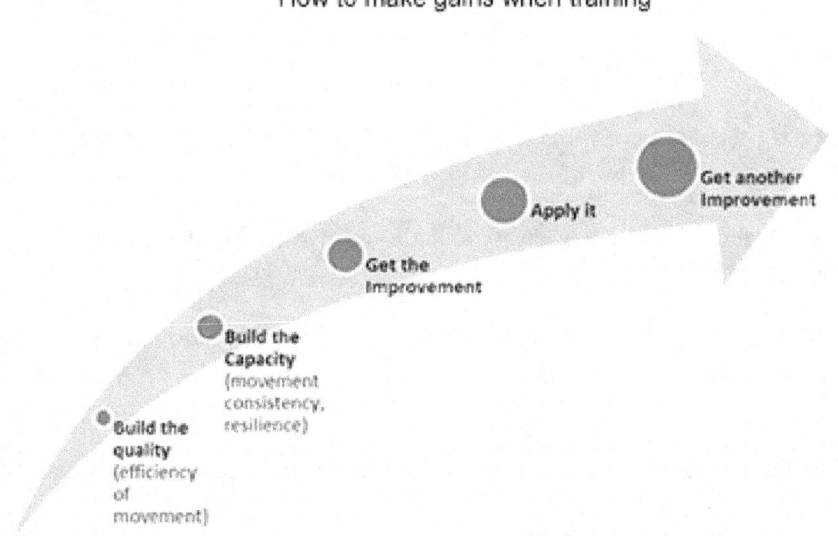

Build upon quality work

Why Pre-Season Training Needs to be Turned on its Head.

Do you start your pre-season with an endurance fitness test? Your players turn up and do either the bleep test or the yo-yo test.

You then train them for a few weeks doing lots of endurance running and retest them before the season starts.

Is this interesting, relevant or fun?

Or are you just gathering random numbers?

I used to do exactly this. When I started working with London Welsh RFC 20 years ago. My plan was this:

1. Test the players

2. Develop an aerobic base.

3. Build up into intermittent endurance work with strength training.

4. Finish the last 2 weeks with speed training.

5. Re-test the players

I checked this plan with some 'expert physiologists' at Brunel University: they thought it was a good plan.

Of course, they did: in a laboratory situation, this would look good as I was training for the test.

Over the last 10 years, working with hundreds of athletes I now realise that the situation should be reversed.

As an athlete, I hated getting tested if I didn't get the feedback, if I didn't think it would help me fight better, or if there was no follow-up training plan to help me improve.

Get Fitter, Faster and Stronger in Pre-season.

As a coach you want your team to be Fitter, Faster and Stronger. But fit for what? You want them on the pitch ready to train and ready to thrive in competition when the season starts.

So, I look at developing 3 qualities:

1. Efficiency: Get them moving well and with control

2. Robustness: Get them able to do that under load, faster, further or heavier.

3. Resilience Get them able to sustain that quality of movement or load for longer.

Who wants to practice bad running, bad lifting, slow agility and irrelevant skill patterns? It is demotivating as a player and a waste of your precious Coaching time as a Coach.

How to Start Pre-season Training.

Testing and evaluation are an important part of pre-season. But just telling players to run further or run faster to improve their test scores may only reinforce their bad technique, and could lead to injury.

My overriding consideration as a Coach is to give the players the tools to do the job.

Choose your tests carefully. If you are in a team field or court sport like Football, Hockey, Rugby or Basketball then the bleep test or yo-yo tests are relevant to the demands of the game. More so than a 1500m or 5km running (or even worse rowing) test to assess your endurance (more test detail here).

But, understand that these tests measure more than endurance. They measure your ability to: accelerate, brake and change direction. All of which are needed in your sports. An example can be seen in this video (https://rb.gy/tpkth6).

So, in conjunction with one of those tests, your first week would be well spent assessing the players' ability to control their bodies.

My motto is '*Little things, done well, consistently.*' If the players are given the tools to do the job, they gain confidence and progress accordingly. You have 6-12 weeks to get players fit, you have to ask yourself:

Are you making them better, or just making them tired?

If your players can accelerate and change direction faster, are strong enough to handle the braking forces when stopping and have a higher top speed, they will improve their test scores.

You can then work on doing more quality movements with a shorter rest time: this will then lead to an improved work capacity.

Most importantly, they will be able to transfer those fitness qualities to the Game where it counts.

50: COACHING WEIGHTLIFTING FOR JUNIORS

Few things in coaching are as rewarding as helping a young person achieve something for the first time: a forward roll, a cartwheel, leaping over a hurdle or standing up with a weight above their head. Their enthusiasm is contagious. Conversely, few things in coaching are as difficult as coaching a group of young people whose minds and bodies are going through the turmoil of puberty and school and socialisation.

We coach children, not weightlifters.

It is easy to get caught up in the frenzy of which foreign programme you follow (German Volume Training, Bulgarian Split Squats, Romanian Deadlifts and Russian Squat Series) and forget that we are coaching children. At our club, we run weightlifting sessions for juniors aged 13-17 (some of our track and field sessions include resistance training but rarely with the barbell). The 13-year-old is an arbitrary figure that I chose based on emotional maturity and that children of that age tend to choose what activities they want to do rather than be told by their parents.

Within this group, we have the obvious difference of boys and girls as well as different physiological ages, training ages and backgrounds and personalities. The younger girls are also learning to manage exercise around their periods and this changes both their mood and ability to lift weights. What seems like the dream child with perfect technique and manners one week can turn into someone who is weaker, less coordinated and doesn't mind slamming the weights around in frustration the next. We have to understand this and be empathetic to these children who are trying to navigate their way through their changing bodies.

Parents will also know that the mood of their child depends on what kind of day they have had at school and what they ate/ drank.

All of the above means that I have to nurture and encourage and support the child before I try to predict what they are going to lift. The totals will fluctuate from session to session: as long as they are safe and enjoy the training they will come back and lift again. The totals will come with time.

Where to start.

I never start with the barbell. I get the children moving in different directions unloaded: lunging, squatting and doing our basic athletic development sequences that connect the hip to shoulder. I can then add a stick to a sequence like the multi-directional lunges

Moving whilst holding an implement above the head is often a novel experience: it raises the person's centre of gravity (COG). Controlling their new body with its new COG is hard enough with just a stick. It also helps develop their shoulder and hip mobility.

I then use dumbbell complexes to prepare the children for lifting. It is easier to get into the positions with lighter weights and they can do the higher repetitions necessary for their learning.

An example would be:

High Pull Snatch

Rotational Press

Hinge (good morning)

Bent over row

Squat.

They do 6-8 repetitions and 2-6 sets. As we progress through the weeks they add sets, up to 6, and then reduce sets once they start to lift the barbell competently until we remove the dumbbells completely.

It is in this stage that the children are learning and building confidence in the new environment. The volume builds strength in small doses. The load is determined by movement competency (as it is for all the lifts): 'smooth' and 'full range'.

Teaching the lifts.

If you take your child to football training they will want to kick the ball and score a goal. It might not look pretty but they have a go. The same applies in weightlifting: I let them have a go. Unlike football, the children have not grown up surrounded by weightlifting and being familiar with the terminology. They aren't allowed to lift free weights in their schools (but are allowed to attempt 1RMs on leg extension machines!) so every technical term is new to them.

I show them the lift first and let them attempt it with a stick or slosh pipe. Our club members who have come through gymnastics and athletics can use the 10kg bar: they have an idea already and are strong enough. We have 10kg,

15kg and 17.5kg bars at our club, as well as the men's 20kg bars. I have seen many school and university gyms that only have 20kg, mostly power, bars. This is discriminatory if you have females who want/ need to lift. Lighter bars are essential for the juniors to learn safely.

After a couple of sets of what ends up as a combination of reverse curls, upright rows and back extensions, I tell the children to put the weights down and watch me break it down in more detail. By trying it out they have already got a 'feel' or perception of what is involved. They have a destination in mind when they now do the sub-components.

They can do these parts of the lift with the 10kg bar and pull from below the knee at first. The combinations of moves could be:

Hinge (good morning)

Behind head press

Overhead Squat.

This helps them get a straight back, control the weight above their head and then get into the bottom position of the snatch. Progression onto the next stage is dependent on competence.

Power snatch (1 rep, ugly looking, to get the weight up)

Press into overhead squat x 3

Snatch Balance x 3

Sotts Press from the bottom x 3-5 (grimacing and moaning about their shoulders, so they usually come up to a parallel squat).

Rest

Repeat.

This might be enough on day one: no heavy loading, lots of repetitions in these novel positions and gaining familiarity with the terminology. I would then go back to the stick/slosh pipe and let them attempt the whole snatch again and praise them on how much better it is looking: invariably it is. **Building on the foundation.**

Observant readers will have noticed that I haven't touched the clean and jerk yet. There are two reasons why I don't start with that combination:

The sequence of two lifts frazzles their brains. The children often combine the two moves into a hybrid split clean that has me reaching for the defibrillator. They need to learn them one at a time before combining them.

The clean is too easy to 'muscle up' at the start. They can use their farm boy/girl strength to get it up and lean back from the waist. Once they start doing this it is hard to stop them. They can't do this in the snatch so they learn to use their legs and back first.

The jerk is hard for the children to learn. I get them practising the foot patterns on the platform and feeling where their legs should land. Then they can attempt it with dumbbells (they are less likely to hit their chin). The dumbbells are harder to control but lighter. Once they get the timing and the control of the landing position they can attempt the lift with the bar.

Over the next few weeks, we repeat what we did in the first session but add in the lifts from the hang and later from the floor. The speed and range of motion of the barbell work are stimuli that create adaptation without the need for extra disks: here my my emphasis is on keeping the bar close to the body and getting under it. We have wooden disks that weigh 0.75kg on either side of the 10kg bar so they can lift from the floor with only 11.5kg at the start. This is too light for some, the bar flies up, so we use the 15kg bars.

Getting the balance between work/range/technique/speed is hard. The children get the 'work' from the dumbbell complexes: they need to feel that they have done something. Developing strength throughout the range of motion required in weightlifting takes time. The muscles adapt to simple loading quickly: bodyweight and dumbbell squats and lunges are great for this. The connective tissues in the shoulders, wrists, hips, ankles and t-spine take longer to adapt and so there is a lag between the 'dumb' strength and the weightlifting totals.

Summary.

Patience and empathy are essential when coaching juniors. They can make rapid progress in their lifts from a low base and it is tempting to pile on weights each week to get a p.b. My aim is not to create a world champion at 13 years old but to get the children competent, confident and enthusiastic about lifting. If they are smiling and tired when they leave they are more likely to come back the next week and then the next. And that is how we create good weightlifters.

51: EXERCISE AS MEDICINE

The words 'High' and 'Performance' are often linked within sporting environments. Unfortunately, they are sometimes used around children and teenagers who have yet to develop sound exercise habits.

The young athletes may play a lot of sports and get selected for county, regional and even national squads based on their skill, experience and parents' willingness to chauffeur and pay, but that is different from being healthy and fit.

Thirty years ago, when studying for my American College of Sports Medicine (ACSM) Health and Fitness Instructor's Certificate, I was told that health comes before fitness comes before performance. This message seems to have been lost somewhere along the way.

Perhaps it got cast aside on the fast track?
(Ahem, I'll see myself out).

Whilst the research quoted below applies to adults (i.e. parents, p.e. teachers and sports coaches) we need to encourage children to get into good habits so they become healthy adults.

If our p.e. syllabi were geared up to physical health and fitness rather than competitive sport, then we might have a chance of creating a healthy nation.

What is healthy exercise?

It is often said that 'exercise is medicine' yet a recent report showed that health practitioners are often uncertain as to what constitutes adequate prescription. If it were a pill, the practitioners would know the dosage, the frequency, weight and duration. For the general population, ideas are even more vague: what is high intensity? what is a MET?

I shall explain a few guidelines and give specific examples as to what that looks like to Joe Public. Specific prescriptions have been shown to have more efficacy.

In a recent review of research studies looking at exercise interventions to improve health, one thing stood out: how unclear the exercise prescriptions were!

Academic studies need to be thoroughly referenced, their statistics have to be sound and they should be reviewed by peers. Yet, when it comes to describing the details of exercises, there is less rigour.

This is frustrating for both other researchers who are looking to replicate the study and to practitioners like Doctors, Physical Therapists and fitness instructors who want to know how much, how often and what type of exercise is most effective.

The good news is that exercise improves not only a person's fitness but also reduces their chance of suffering from non-communicable diseases as demonstrated in these two studies:

1. Improved Cardio Respiratory Fitness reduces the chance of all Cardiovascular Disease and Cancer Muscle (https://rb.gy/3ti03k).

2. Muscle-strengthening exercises reduce the risk of Cardiovascular Diseases, total cancer, diabetes and lung cancer, as well as improving musculoskeletal health (https://rb.gy/wup5f1).

The evidence is clear: exercising to improve your cardiorespiratory fitness or doing muscle-strengthening exercises reduces your chance of suffering from non-communicable diseases and some cancers.

How much Exercise Medicine should I prescribe?

This is the tricky part. For the habitual exercisers, those who do something every week, the message is simple: Keep it up.

It is important to understand how difficult it is for people to change their behaviour, especially if they lack motivation, confidence, capacity or understanding. That is why we need to encourage and reward existing behaviour and build from there.

The keen cyclist, runner, dancer, walker and swimmer might benefit from doing some muscle-strengthening exercises. This is best done in their environment to start rather than tell them to 'join a gym' which requires overcoming a whole different set of obstacles.

Examples include:
Bodyweight exercises before or after their current workouts.
· Sit to stands (squats) and step-ups on park benches.
· Inclined press-ups on the park bench and tricep dips (or poolside).
· Lunges and standing jumps before setting off.
· Carrying the bicycle at arm's length in various positions.

The evidence is that an hour a week of muscle-strengthening exercises reduces the risk of disease, but more than that doesn't reduce the risk further. For those who aren't doing these types of exercises, little and often is as good as visiting the gym once a week.

The size of the weight doesn't matter, it's the frequency and habit that counts.

The keen gym user who only lifts weights will benefit from some cardiorespiratory type exercises. Something that gets them out of breath or raises their heart rate for a sustained time. For this group, this could be integrated into their gym session: they are already there. This could be used in the warm-up, or after lifting their weights. Stationary cycling, jumping rope and treadmill running are all suitable.

For the sedentary person, building confidence is the key. Encouraging them to do a little bit more will allow them to achieve success. For them, telling them they need to do an hour of muscle-strengthening exercises each week is as hard to conceive as asking me to climb Mount Everest: I would not know where to start.

The same applies to cardiorespiratory exercises: the sedentary person will be intimidated by the current recommendation that:

"All healthy adults aged 18–65 yr should participate in moderate-intensity aerobic physical activity for a minimum of 30 minutes on five days per week, or vigorous-intensity aerobic activity for a minimum of 20 minutes on three days per week."
Physical Activity Guidelines Resources (acsm.org)

Instead, if they are encouraged to do a little bit more, then they will improve. No, this won't meet the guidelines, but it is an improvement. Think of a snowball rolling down a mountain: it starts with a tiny golf ball size and accumulates more and more.

For this population, doing more in the home and work is a great place to start. This can include:
· Parking further away from the office, supermarket, cinema, and restaurant.
· Using stairs rather than elevators.
· Using the bathroom on a different level from the one you work on (also works at home, go up and down the stairs each time you need to use the bathroom, make a drink, eat a snack, check social media on your phone).
· Walk around the block in the morning, lunchtime and evening.
· Cleaning the house more frequently or tidying up the gardening.

Once this person has got into these tiny habits, they can think about doing longer walks, getting a walking buddy, and taking up an active hobby such as line-dancing or bowling.

Summary.

The good news is that exercise improves health, this is indisputable. The bad news is that no one dose suits every individual. Instead, health practitioners should seek to understand where the person is now and encourage more exercises in that environment and build from there.

52: WHAT IS THE END GAME FOR YOUR YOUNG ATHLETE?

The Marvel Movie Avengers: End Game smashed all box office records when it was released five years ago. The Marvel Cinematic Universe (MCU) which started with Iron Man in 2008 and has encompassed 21 previous movies was wrapped up in this three-hour epic. Multiple plot lines, dozens of characters, cameos and references to past movies were included. Nothing like this had ever been done before. Eleven years beforehand no one predicted this.

Yet, if we look back at the lead-up to End Game, it seems ordered and sequential.

Start small with individual movies and add little post-credit scenes that act as a teaser for the next film. Slowly add more characters and finish in a big epic four years later: Avengers Assemble.

Phew, that was exciting.

Now dig deeper into the Marvel Canon, take a risk on the lesser-known Guardians of the Galaxy, build up to a second Avengers movie and use existing plots like Civil War to use lots more characters. Now the cash is rolling in, we have a loyal fan base. Let's try digging deeper to add minority characters like Black Panther and Captain Marvel. Those movies were even bigger hits, earning more money than Spiderman and Doctor Strange.

In 2008 if you had said that a movie with a black character as the lead or a superhero movie with a female lead would earn more than a Spiderman movie, you would have been laughed at. These things were not "givens"; risks and luck played a part.

DC have tried to create their version of the MCU but failed miserably and with considerable expense.

What's this got to do with young athletes?

Sports' National Governing Bodies (NGBs) in the UK offer 'pathways' to the International Stage, predicting success in 10 years. There is simply no evidence that a single route will lead to success.

Copying one person's route to the top is unlikely to succeed: just as DC have failed to reproduce what Marvel did with End Game.

Just because it worked once, doesn't mean it will work again, even in the same environment: Disney has spectacularly failed to produce the quality of this movie tie-in epic since. No one could predict this, either.

Todd Rosen in his excellent book, **The End of Average**, says this about pathways (1):

"We presume the best way to be successful in life is to follow that well-blazed trail. But what the pathways principle tells us is that we are always creating our own pathway for the first time, inventing it as we go along, since every decision we make- or every event we experience- changes the possibilities available to us." (p139).

How then can we help develop athletes to become champions?

This is the wrong question for club coaches, parents and teachers.

To produce champions at 22-26 we need many people participating in physical activity, every child sampling several sports over their primary and secondary school years and then competition. The best people will emerge from 16-19 years old and then the NGBs can tailor elite-level training to those few who show capability and desire (rather than those whose parents can afford fuel and coaching).

To paraphrase Owen Slot in **The Talent Lab,** *"UK sport is all about the shop window of Olympic medals, but we don't have enough people in the shop."*(2).

The question I ask as a parent is:

How can I help my children develop various physical skills in a fun and challenging environment?

This is what I look for when choosing activities for my children.

In their primary school years, horse riding, lifeguarding, climbing in our local area have been led by excellent people and have included a mix of fun, skill and challenge. At no point have I been asked or asked about 'talent' and competition. I realise that by keeping moving and being exposed to different environments my children will develop in ways that I can't imagine or foresee, or control.

The observant reader will have noticed that the three activities I mentioned could be classed as individual 'sports'. Excelsior Athletic Development Club offers gymnastics, athletics and weight lifting, 3 more 'individual' sports.

Except for horse riding which is a 1 adult: 1 child ratio, all of the other activities happen in group environments. Collaboration is essential- belaying a fellow climber, rescuing a drowning victim or supporting a handspring all require another person to help.

The children compete like crazy sometimes in these sessions- who can get up the wall fastest, who can hurdle the fastest or throw the furthest, who can hold a headstand for the longest. But, not every child is trying to beat another person. The competition is self-organised for the most part. I always put some competitive element in each session- either a challenge to themselves- or against each other.

This is different from the team sport environments that I have witnessed for the under 10s, where the emphasis is on winning on Saturday or Sunday and the weekly training reflects this. Do the children want a weekly match against other teams? Or are they thrust into the environment and get swept along for the ride?

More importantly, children are simply too young to understand the group dynamics of team sports. They focus on one thing- themselves. This was well known in the past in physical education circles, where team sports were not introduced until about 10-11 years old in schools (1,2). Unfortunately, the commercialisation of youth sports has not meant a corresponding increase in understanding of what activity is best for the child's age and stage of development.

My son and daughter both represented their Primary school in team events. The matches were few and far between, enough for a taster, not enough to be a grind. They had developed the basic skills of throwing, catching, striking, running and jumping that allowed them to pick up sport-specific skills when shown.

Compare that to the girls I saw this week doing cricket who flinched away when a ball was thrown underarm to them from 2 metres away. Cricket is a prime example of a sport that expresses skill rather than develops skill. When there is one ball and 22 players, how much time can be spent getting better by playing a match?

Where then to start?

Start where the child is now, not where a model says they should be. One of the biggest changes in my coaching over the last 10 years is using guided discovery at the younger ages rather than directions.

In gymnastics, the forward roll is often used as a benchmark of achievement.

In this video you can see me learning from a gymnastics coach, with everything returning to the forward roll (https://rb.gy/iz9bu3).

In this video you can see me leading the boys and allowing them to work out different movements (https://rb.gy/7555ss).

They may or may not be able to perform a forward roll at the end of this session, but that is not the aim. The aim is to get them to learn and explore how their body works. If they feel competent, have learnt something and had the chance to try new ways of doing something themselves, they are more likely to return. Keeping them involved is critical.

Good coaches know this already. But, if you are trying to "fun it up" with 5-year-olds trying to learn rugby with a ball bigger than their heads, you are unlikely to succeed. You are trying to get them to adapt to a system for which they are unprepared: physically, socially, emotionally and skill-wise.

By piecing together adult-led initiatives and reverse engineering from the Olympics into the youth system, you are more likely to create the next Aquaman rather than the next Iron Man.

References.

1. The end of average. Todd Rose. Harper One (2016).

2. The Talent Lab: The secrets of creating and sustaining success. Owen Slot. Ebury Press (2017).

3. Physical Education for children: A focus on the teaching process. Ed. B. Logsdon. Lea & Febiger (1977).

4. Movement: Physical Education in the Primary years. Department of Education and Science. HMSO (1972).

ABOUT THE AUTHOR

James Marshall is the Head Coach of Excelsior Athletic Development Club. (Instagram: @excelsioradclub)

He has an MSc in Sports Coaching, and is a qualified coach in Athletics, Gymnastics and Weightlifting. He is a certified strength and conditioning coach, and spent ten years working in health and fitness prior to that.

He is a 4th Dan in Shotokan Karate and competed in the Shoto World Cup in 2004. He is a Masters Weightlifter, winning British titles in 2022-24, came second in the 2023 European Championships and has qualified for the World Championships in Finland in 2024.

His debut novel, The Poster, was runner-up in the 2023/24 Pen to Print Book Challenge.